NCT Book of
Antenatal Tests

NCT Book of Antenatal Tests

Mary Nolan

Thorsons

An Imprint of HarperCollins*Publishers*
in collaboration with National Childbirth Trust Publishing

While the author of this work has made every effort to ensure that the information contained in this book is as accurate and up to date as possible at the time of publication, medical and pharmaceutical knowledge is constantly changing and the application of it to particular circumstances depends on many factors. Therefore it is recommended that readers always consult a qualified medical specialist for individual advice. This book should not be used as an alternative to seeking specialist medical advice, which should be sought before any action is taken. The author and publishers cannot be held responsible for any errors and omissions that may be found in the text, or any actions that may be taken by a reader as a result of any reliance on the information contained in the text, which is taken entirely at the reader's own risk.

Thorsons/National Childbirth Trust Publishing
Thorsons is an Imprint of HarperCollins*Publishers*
77–85 Fulham Palace Road
Hammersmith, London W6 8JB

Published by Thorsons and
National Childbirth Trust Publishing 1998

1 3 5 7 9 10 8 6 4 2

© NCT Publishing 1998

Mary Nolan asserts the moral right to
be identified as the author of this work

A catalogue record for this book
is available from the British Library

ISBN 0 7225 3604 6

Printed and bound in Great Britain by
Caledonian International Book Manufacturing Ltd, Glasgow

Contents

Acknowledgements

I would first and foremost like to acknowledge the insights offered me by all the women to whom I have spoken about antenatal testing. Their stories, which are at the heart of this book, taught me more than I could have learned in any other way. During the course of my research for the book, I made contact with a variety of voluntary organizations and was impressed by the enthusiasm and professionalism with which they met my requests for information – organizations such as the National Childbirth Trust, the Down's Syndrome Association, REACH, the Cystic Fibrosis Trust, The Terrence Higgins Trust and Positively Women. Finally, there are certain individuals whom I would like to mention by name for their very special contributions, both in terms of the time they gave me and the generosity with which they shared their experiences; these are Pauline Kell, Professor Martin Whittle, Deborah Gough, Ruth Kirchmeier and Susan Clydesdale-Cotter. I would also like to thank Sandy Oliver, Joanna Hawthorne and Helen Stathan for reading and commenting on the manuscript.

Introduction

After the first excitement of finding out that you are pregnant is over, it's quite natural to feel anxious from time to time, or perhaps all the time, about whether your baby will be healthy. Everyone likes to think that their child will be able to join in all the sporting and educational activities which are available to children today, and that he or she will not be prevented from doing so because of physical or mental ill health. Very often, the parents of a disabled child find themselves pitied because other people see only the disappointment and difficulties of having a child who is different from other children. It's hard for 'normal' parents of 'normal' children to appreciate that there can be any joy in parenting a disabled child. Our society does not find it easy to accept people with a disability although great strides in recognizing and catering for their needs have been made in recent years.

It could be argued that there is no such thing as 'the perfect baby'. Perfect babies are an advertising dream – only babies in adverts never cry, never have dirty nappies, never have cradle cap and never get their mothers and fathers up in the middle of the night! Every baby is an individual and will have some individual peculiarity which marks him out from other children as he grows up. He may be hyperactive or allergic to penicillin, or he may be dyslexic, or asthmatic or suffer from eczema or have an irrational fear of lifts or plug holes.

All our children have health problems which, you could say, means that they're not 'perfect', but parents learn to live with these problems and help their children to manage them. Because it is now possible to test unborn babies for a wide range of mental and physical conditions, we have perhaps lost sight of the fact that there is still no such thing as 'the perfect baby' and probably never will be.

Of course, there is a difference between caring for a child who has eczema and one who has Down's Syndrome. Eczema will probably not rule the child's life (or her parents') in the same way that having serious learning difficulties will. Nobody except the parents of an unborn baby can decide what kinds of health problems they could cope with in their child and what kinds of problems would overstretch their physical, emotional and financial resources. Some parents don't consider that there's any decision to make. For moral or religious reasons, they feel that they have no right to end a pregnancy. They are prepared to accept, love and care for their child whether he or she is normal or poorly or disabled. Other parents feel unwilling to bring a baby into the world who may have to endure a lot of suffering. They feel that the stress of caring, day in and day out for a child with a serious physical or mental disability would destroy the quality of their own lives and that of other children they may already have.

Antenatal tests can now tell parents more about their unborn baby than it has ever been possible to know before. However, some parents feel that the information tests provide is too complicated to be useful in helping them make decisions, and therefore choose not to have any tests at all. Some parents agree to have a test without properly understanding what the test is for or what further decisions they might have to make if the result is positive. Some parents really research the tests and are clear in their own minds about what they would do if their baby was found to have a problem. It's important to remember that tests are not there to help doctors make decisions about what is best for you or your baby, but to help you make those decisions.

One of the most important issues raised by antenatal testing is how much information parents are given before they have any tests and how much support they receive while they are having them. This concern is expressed by women such as Jemma and Nikki:

'I am unhappy that the technology for screening has far outstripped any counselling available. I dislike the assumption that screening and therefore the willingness to abort should be considered the norm. Much media attention is focused on the ethics of IVF but hardly any on antenatal screening which is much more common. The issue made my pregnancies very unhappy.'

Jemma

'I was given no information about testing when I became pregnant. My local hospital telephoned me on a Saturday afternoon to tell me my triple test result was high risk for Down's Syndrome and would I go in the following Monday for an amniocentesis. I did not even know who was on the other end of the phone.'

Nikki

This book aims to give information to help you make your own choices about antenatal testing. It doesn't suggest that one choice is better than another, but it is based on the principle that no one should be asked to make decisions which could affect the rest of their lives without having all the information they need.

Why Have Any Tests?

Reassurance

The first thing to say is that you don't have to have any antenatal tests. Some people think the tests are compulsory. They're not! The decision about which tests to have and how many tests is entirely yours, although in some circumstances you may have to travel to a different hospital and possibly pay to have a test that is not on offer locally. You may decide that you would like to have a test because if the results are normal (which they nearly always are) you will feel very reassured and be more relaxed during the rest of your pregnancy. However, some parents think they will be reassured by favourable results and then find that they go on being anxious. Having the tests makes them focus on all the things which could be wrong with their baby and they lose sight of the much greater likelihood that their baby will be fine:

> 'The scan is quite anxiety-provoking. I mean it's nice, too, but I found both mine quite anxiety-provoking. What the doctor said worried me, and what she didn't say, and I was worrying what she was looking at and all the rest of it.'

> *Ciara*

Preparing for the Birth of a Sick or Disabled Baby

You may decide that you want to find out if your baby is going to have a health problem so that you have time to prepare yourself as thoroughly as possible. This was Donna's reason:

'I told my midwife that I would be unprepared to abort. I had a blood test for Down's/spina bifida but only so I could be prepared at the birth if there were any special needs.'

Donna

You might feel that the shock of giving birth to a baby with, for example a cleft lip and palate, will be very much less if you already know about the problem and that you will be able to enjoy the birth more if you are prepared beforehand.

It might also be very useful to know while you are still pregnant if your baby has a serious health problem so that you can make a decision with your doctor about where to give birth. You can choose a hospital which has a Special Care Baby Unit so that your baby can immediately receive the very best care available rather than having to be transferred from a hospital which hasn't got highly specialized facilities.

Choosing a Termination

You may be very clear in your own mind that you want to have tests while you are pregnant because if your baby has a serious condition such as spina bifida or Down's Syndrome, you will choose a termination:

'I was prepared to have an amniocentesis because I felt that if I had a Down's child, that would be the end of my life, my work, and my marriage probably; and I didn't want to have one because I've seen two or three people with Down's children whose lives have fallen apart.'

Jacinta

You may well find excellent support from health staff if you have to make the difficult decision to end your pregnancy:

> 'We were seen by a very caring and sympathetic sister and consultant obstetrician with whom we made arrangements for the termination to go ahead.'

Amy
(SATFA News, *March 1997*)

Some parents choose not to have any antenatal testing because they feel strongly that to end a pregnancy by having a termination is wrong. Their convictions help them to carry on with their pregnancy even if it is confirmed that their baby has a serious medical condition which will affect the whole of his or her life. However, some women and couples who have strong religious ideals and practise their faith devoutly, may feel that, under certain circumstances, their conscience allows them to make a decision which ministers of their church might not approve of.

Sometimes, women say that they have been told they can only have a particular test such as chorionic villus sampling or amniocentesis if they agree to end their pregnancy should their baby prove to have Down's Syndrome or some other serious disabling condition. This kind of pressure is unethical. However, it's not uncommon as the following accounts suggest:

> 'The midwife advised us not to have an amniocentesis unless we were sure we would terminate the pregnancy if there was something wrong with the baby. We were shocked by this.'

Lucy

'My GP, while supporting my wish to have the chorionic villus sampling test, assumed termination of the pregnancy was my only option had the results been positive for a chromosomal abnormality.'

Shaheeda

'We felt we would be supported if we chose to have a termination, but not really if we went ahead with the pregnancy.'

Anya

You should never be put under any pressure to have a termination if the result of a test confirms that your baby has a serious health problem. Write to the General Manager of the Maternity Unit if anyone tries to force your hand in this way.

Special Circumstances

If you already have a child who has Down's Syndrome or spina bifida, you may feel that you want to be certain that the baby you are now pregnant with does not. If you have a child with a rare genetic disorder or have given birth to a baby who died of a genetic abnormality, you will understandably feel very anxious about the baby you are now carrying. Today, it is possible to do pregnancy tests for a huge range of genetic conditions and you should be offered these tests if you already have one affected child or if you come from a family where there is someone affected or if you have the condition yourself. If this is your situation, ask your GP to refer you to the Clinical Genetics Unit at the Regional Referral Centre where there will be professionals with particular expertise in helping parents like yourself make decisions about antenatal testing.

If you are disabled, you might have strong feelings about the possibility of having a disabled baby. You might feel that you simply couldn't look after a child with special needs on top of managing your own daily life as a disabled person. It might, therefore, be particularly important for you to have diagnostic tests in order to be as certain as possible that your baby is healthy. You, too, should have the chance to discuss your situation with a midwife or counsellor specially trained in helping people make decisions about antenatal tests.

Getting to Grips with the Tests: Screening Tests and Diagnostic Tests

The first thing to understand about antenatal tests is that some are SCREENING and some are DIAGNOSTIC.

Screening Tests Are:

- the nuchal translucency test for Down's Syndrome which you can have when you are about 10–12 weeks pregnant
- blood tests which are normally offered to you when you are about 16–18 weeks pregnant
- ultrasound scans (although these can sometimes be diagnostic)

Diagnostic Tests Are:

- chorionic villus sampling
- amniocentesis
- ultrasound scans (although these are sometimes only for screening)

A screening test cannot tell you for certain that your baby either has or has not got a particular condition such as spina bifida or Down's Syndrome. It only tells you what your risk is of having a baby with that condition.

A diagnostic test should tell you *for certain* if your baby has a particular condition.

SCREENING TEST
A screening test tells you what your risk is of having a baby with Down's Syndrome or spina bifida.

DIAGNOSTIC TEST
A diagnostic test tells you for certain whether your baby has Down's Syndrome or spina bifida (or some other serious condition).

Screening tests are generally the first to be offered to a pregnant woman because they are easy to perform and do not carry any risk of miscarriage.

Diagnostic tests are more complicated and more expensive and, in the case of chorionic villus sampling, cordocentesis and amniocentesis, carry a small risk that the mother will have a miscarriage as a result of the procedure.

Even the results of a diagnostic test may not be 100 per cent reliable. Every now and then, you will read in the newspapers about the results of tests being mixed up. One woman is told at 24 weeks of pregnancy that her baby is fine although he is born four months later with Down's Syndrome; another is told that her baby has Down's Syndrome, chooses a termination and at the postmortem, the baby is discovered to be normal. Although these instances are very rare, they do occur and it's important to remember that there are no absolute certainties when it comes to antenatal testing.

Understanding Risk

When you get the results of a *screening* test, you will be told that you are either 'screen negative' or 'screen positive'. Screen negative means that your risk of having a baby with the condition being tested for is less than 1 in 250 (or perhaps less than 1 in 300 depending on the cut-off point used by the laboratory that analyses your blood sample). Your risk therefore is very small indeed. It might be 1 in 480 in which case you might compare it to thinking of a number between 1 and 480 and asking a friend to guess the number you are thinking of. If she made 480 guesses, she would be wrong 479 times and right only once. She's far more likely not to guess your number than to guess it.

If you are told you are screen positive, your risk of having a baby with the condition being tested for is higher than 1 in 250. For example, it might be 1 in 150 or 1 in 40. This means that the likelihood of your baby being healthy is still infinitely greater than the chances of her having a problem but you have a higher risk than a woman who has received a screen negative result.

People's natural reaction to a screen positive result is to think immediately that their baby must have a problem. Perhaps we all have a tendency to catastrophize! But even if your risk is estimated at 1 in 4 for Down's Syndrome or spina bifida, this still means that you are three times more likely to have a healthy baby than you are to have a disabled baby.

Sometimes it's helpful to 'see' how big the risk is. Here's what a screen negative result with a risk of 1 in 500 looks like on graph paper and a screen positive result of 1 in 40:

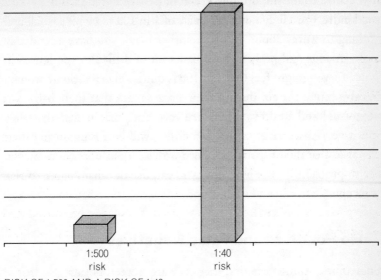

RISK OF 1:500 AND A RISK OF 1:40

What kind of risk people find acceptable will vary from one person to the next. If, for example, you already have a child with a disability and are sure that you could not cope with another highly dependent child, you might consider a risk of 1 in 100 for Down's to be very high and choose to have a diagnostic test to find out for certain whether your baby is affected. On the other hand, if you have been trying for a baby for years and are told that the baby you are now carrying has a 1 in 100 chance of Down's Syndrome, you might decide that this is an acceptable risk. You don't want to have a diagnostic test because there is a small chance that you might have a miscarriage afterwards. For you, the possible risks of a diagnostic test are less acceptable than living with the knowledge that there is a small chance that your baby will be born with Down's Syndrome.

The way in which people interpret risk is very much influenced by their personality and the kind of experiences they have had in life.

If you are a confident, optimistic sort of person and life has dealt with you kindly, you might consider a risk of 1 in 100 to be very small and nothing to worry about. If, on the other hand, you have a tendency to be anxious and perhaps have had a lot of difficult experiences in your life, you might feel that 1 in 100 is quite a big risk. Some women are absolutely certain during their pregnancies that their baby will be normal and healthy; others are constantly frightened that they will have a miscarriage or that something will go wrong during their labour or that their baby will be born with a serious physical or mental health problem. In the end, only you can decide what degree of risk is acceptable to you and what is not.

False Positives and False Negatives

Sometimes, women are told that they are 'screen negative' – that is that their risk of having a baby with Down's Syndrome is less than 1 in 250 – but still give birth to a baby who has Down's Syndrome. A 'screen negative' result does not mean that a baby definitely hasn't got Down's, but many parents interpret it as such. The shock of then giving birth to an affected baby is probably far greater than it would have been if they had never had any tests done at all. Perhaps the strongest objection to antenatal screening is that it may lull parents into a false sense of security about their baby's well-being or, if they receive a 'screen positive' result, make them terribly anxious for the whole of their pregnancy until finally, in the vast majority of cases, they give birth to a perfectly healthy baby. The emotional impact of screening tests has been widely researched, but listening to parents tell their stories suggests that there can often be a heavy price to pay.

Occasionally, very tragic situations occur when a woman receives a 'false positive' result. She is told that her baby is at high risk of Down's Syndrome and makes the decision to have an amniocentesis to obtain a diagnosis. The amniocentesis then causes a miscarriage:

'I was not given any counselling about the Alphafeto Protein (AFP) test which I accepted as routine. I was twenty weeks pregnant when I was told that, although I was only 26, I had the risk of a woman of 37 of having a Down's baby. The amniocentesis was booked for the next day, so I had no time at all to think it over and in any case, I was on my own and in a state of extreme anxiety. I had the amnio on Tuesday and the following Friday I started getting pains which I now know were the beginning of labour. I was admitted to hospital that night and gave birth to a little girl six hours later. I was not informed of the results of the amnio until I rang up the hospital and was told that the baby had been normal. This was all nearly four years ago and I am still mourning the loss of my daughter who would have been just about ready to go to school now had it not been for the antenatal testing.'

Sylvia

Sylvia's story is the saddest possible outcome of antenatal testing, but it is a fairly rare one. Testing does, however, sometimes lead to the accidental loss of a healthy baby or to the termination of babies who do not have severe health problems. A study carried out from 1990 to 1994 in Yorkshire looked at the accuracy of ultrasound scanning in pregnancy. 354 pregnancies were terminated during the four year period because of serious abnormalities diagnosed by scanning. In 240 cases, the postmortem diagnosis confirmed the scan diagnosis. In 112 cases, the post-mortem diagnosis showed that the babies had more serious problems than the ultrasound scan had suggested, or had additional problems. In two cases, the babies were found to have less severe problems than the ultrasound diagnosis and, had the parents and their professional carers known this, the decision to go ahead with the termination might not have been made.

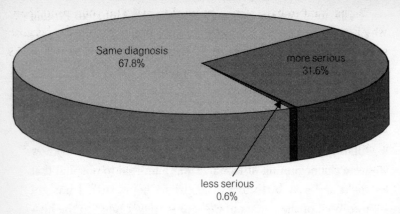

Same diagnosis
67.8%

more serious
31.6%

less serious
0.6%

ACCURACY OF ULTRASOUND:
POSTMORTEM DIAGNOSIS VS SCAN DIAGNOSIS

- ❑ 67.8% pregnancies with same diagnosis at postmortem as at scanning
- ❑ 31.6% pregnancies with more serious diagnoses at postmortem than at scanning
- ❑ 0.6% pregnancies with less serious diagnoses at postmortem than at scanning

Deciding Which Tests to Have

Always remember that you can decide not to have any tests at all during your pregnancy. This is a perfectly reasonable decision and you're quite within your rights to make it. Nobody should put you under any pressure to have tests that you don't want. Many antenatal screening tests are now routine and health professionals are sometimes surprised when women choose not to have them. Don't feel coerced into changing your mind; you know best what is right for you.

If you want to have tests, you need to make up your mind about which ones as soon as you know you are pregnant. This is because some of the tests have to be carried out during the first twelve weeks of pregnancy, well before you have a bump to show!

The timetable for testing looks like this:

test	timing	screening/diagnostic
nuchal translucency	10–13 weeks	screening
chorionic villus sampling	around 11 weeks	diagnostic
amniocentesis	13–18 weeks	diagnostic
ultrasound	8–40 weeks	may be screening or diagnostic
blood tests	16–18 weeks	screening

Getting the Information You Need

You should be given all the information you need in order to decide which tests to have or whether to have any and then to be supported in your decision. Just because you decide not to have any tests doesn't mean that you stop worrying about your baby:

'Once we had told the GP that we would not consider a termination, we were told not to have any screening as it would cause us anxiety and there would be no point to it if we intended to have the baby anyway. While accepting the logic of this, it has caused us some distress as the decision not to have any tests does not in any way reduce our anxiety about having a child with a disability. Some counselling support or at least a little more time from the GP might have been helpful.'

Daphne

It is probably true to say that most parents find antenatal testing stressful, but there's no doubt that being given information, time to think and support helps:

'My community midwife's attitude was excellent. She explained all the options in some detail to my husband and myself during a home visit at 14 weeks; she answered all our questions. She gave us very reassuring advice about how to make sure (if we decided to go ahead with the test) that I saw the consultant himself at my first hospital appointment at 16 weeks in order to discuss the matter with him and arrange for the test to be carried out by him in person.'

Courtney

'The staff involved with the scan were very helpful regarding any questions I had. It would be nice if all pregnant women were given adequate information and support in choices about antenatal care.'

Meg

When you first go to your local surgery to see your GP or midwife about your pregnancy and to discuss what kind of antenatal care you would like and where you want your baby to be born, you can also ask about the various antenatal tests available and how you can arrange to have them. The information your doctor or midwife will give you is quite complicated and it's useful to ask for some leaflets or written information which you can look through at home. There may be a midwife at your local hospital who specializes in counselling women and their families about antenatal testing. Ask your GP or midwife if there is such a person. There are also organizations which you can contact if you want more information. (Addresses are given at the end of this book.) The booklets they produce for pregnant women explain antenatal tests in everyday language rather than medical jargon.

After you have had a first chat with your GP or midwife about testing and thought about what was said, you may feel that you want to talk again. Don't hesitate to make another appointment and, in the meantime, jot down all the questions you want to ask. Everybody has experienced the problem of going to see a health professional and not being able to remember what they wanted to say!

Talk to the important people in your life about whether to have any tests and which ones would be best for you. Your partner needs to share the responsibility for decisions about testing and the two of you need to be in agreement about what you would do if you got a positive result. If you cannot agree, and one of you has to take the initiative in making a decision about testing, you need at least to understand each other's positions.

It's also very helpful to talk to other women about their experiences of antenatal testing. This book contains many quotes from women who have been recently pregnant and have had to make decisions about antenatal tests. They illustrate the huge variety of ideas, motives and feelings which influence the way people handle pregnancy testing. If you want to find out how you might feel about having a test, waiting for the results and then acting on those results, your best source of information will be other women and couples who have been through the experience before you.

Not all the tests described in this book are available on the NHS and not all are available in every part of the country. Even within the same geographical area, hospitals may vary in the tests which they offer to pregnant women. Most women should find that they can have a simple blood test for screening and ultrasound scanning is also available just about everywhere. However, more complicated tests or tests which require very expensive equipment may not be offered to you unless you are over the age of 35 or you specifically ask and you may have to travel to a Regional Referral Centre in order to have them. For example, if you want the nuchal translucency test which is a very good screening test for Down's Syndrome and you don't live in the south east, you may have to travel to London in order to have it. You may also have to pay for the test. Similarly, the mouthwash test which is to see whether parents are carriers of the gene for cystic fibrosis is not generally provided by the NHS and you may have to have the test done privately.

Being Tested

Whether you are going to have a simple blood test or a routine scan or a more complicated test such as chorionic villus sampling or amniocentesis, try to take your partner or your mum or a close friend with you to the hospital to look after you. Sometimes, you are kept waiting quite a while and it's helpful to have another person to share the time with you and perhaps distract you a little.

When you go in for the test, try very hard to relax – even though this is not easy when you are in a clinical environment surrounded by people wearing white coats and perhaps masks. A simple relaxation technique is to focus on your breathing. If your breathing is relaxed, you will be too. When you are breathing normally, your breathing is rhythmical. Your 'in-breath' is perfectly balanced by your 'out-breath'. When people are stressed or panicky, their breathing becomes shallow and they 'catch at' their in-breath and often don't breathe out properly. To keep your breathing rhythmical, concentrate on relaxing each time you breathe out and as you breathe out, let your shoulders drop and feel loose. Think to yourself 'RE' as you breathe in and 'LAX' as you breathe out.

Waiting for Results

Many women are very anxious while they are waiting for their test results and find it difficult to concentrate on their everyday lives. Waiting two to three weeks for the results of an amniocentesis is particularly stressful and your life seems to be 'on hold'. You may try to forget that you are pregnant during this period, or even start to hate your baby because you are so anxious. If the results are favourable and indicate that it is extremely unlikely that your baby has Down's Syndrome or spina bifida or any of the other conditions which the test may have investigated, you will probably feel that a load has fallen off your back:

> 'The scan and CVS [chorionic villus sampling] I had were excellent. I felt very confident that the results would be as accurate as was possible – they gave me the information I wanted and I did not feel the need to seek further reassurance by more tests.'

> *Augusta*

It has to be said, however, that not every woman feels reassured, even by the results of a diagnostic test. In the following quotation, a midwife describes the reaction of one woman for whom she had cared:

'A lady came along and her AFP was slightly low and she had an amniocentesis and everything was fine. But it didn't reassure her; she spent the rest of her pregnancy worrying so, for her, it didn't work.'

If you have a blood test to screen for Down's Syndrome and spina bifida, you may well never get the results of the test if they are screen negative. Most women find the 'no news, good news' system which many hospitals operate extremely unsatisfactory. If it's not good enough for you never to hear the results of your blood test, ring the hospital about 10 days after the test and ask. Just occasionally, women are not told the results of a diagnostic test such as amniocentesis if the results are negative. This is absolutely unforgivable but it does make the point that you need to keep checking with the hospital to see if the results are through.

If your test results show that your baby does have Down's Syndrome or spina bifida or is at high risk of having one of these conditions, your GP or midwife or a doctor from the hospital should ring you and make an appointment to see you, hopefully later the same day. Some GPs and midwives bring the results in person and visit you at home. This represents one end of the spectrum of care, but at the other end of the spectrum, it's not unknown for results to be sent by post and not always first class!

Coping with Bad News

However you felt initially about your pregnancy and even if you didn't really want to be pregnant, you are going to be immensely shocked by the news that your baby has been diagnosed as having a serious problem. It's probably impossible to imagine the depth of emotion which people feel and we can only listen to their descriptions:

'My first reaction as a Christian was to say that we would continue (with the pregnancy) – I had always thought previously that if a baby was still alive, who was I to take that away? But it is so easy to have strong principles when they are not being put to the test. Later at home, my husband and I discussed the problem at length – I found myself praying to have a miscarriage when I had spent the previous 20 weeks praying not to.'

Cicely
(SATFA News, *September 1996*)

To begin with, you may feel that you simply can't believe what you have been told. You are sure there must have been a mistake and that your results have been mixed up with someone else's. It may be impossible for you to accept that the baby whom you have loved and nurtured for several months is not the baby of your dreams, but a baby who has major health problems.

You may feel very angry that this terrible thing has happened to you, and wonder what you have done to deserve such unhappiness:

'We were told our baby had Down's Syndrome. I immediately presumed that it must be because of something I had done during my pregnancy. I wanted to scream that it just wasn't fair and then I cried and cried and cried. And Simon cried.'

Karli

Perhaps you have been trying to have a baby for a long time and just a few weeks after the joy of finding out that you were pregnant comes the news that all is not well. It may seem terribly unfair that other women should have babies so easily, and give birth to two or three who are perfectly healthy, when your precious baby whom you have waited for for such a long time is not healthy.

As the news sinks in, you may simply feel in despair, unable to face your friends, your family or perhaps even your partner. You may feel that life isn't worth living and that everything you had hoped for in the future has been taken away from you at a stroke.

All these are normal reactions. You have suffered a bereavement, the loss of a dream. You have every right to feel angry, helpless, depressed and unable to see your way ahead. Whatever decision you make at this point, you will need to grieve for the baby you had hoped to have and who isn't the baby you are carrying.

Your midwife and doctor may be pressing you to decide what you want to do next. It's a good idea to ask for a day or two so that you can think a little more calmly about what has happened. You may need to have a long cry, to phone your mum, or be close to your partner. If you feel that there is nobody to whom you can talk, remember that there are people working for organizations such as the National Childbirth Trust and SATFA – Support Around Termination For Abnormality – who will be more than willing to listen to you and help you. Do get in touch. Or you might want to contact a minister of your religion to seek guidance and support.

Making Decisions

It may be that antenatal testing will face you with some of the biggest decisions you have ever had to make in your life. Making a decision, for example, about whether to end your pregnancy if your baby is found to have a serious disabling condition is a huge one and whatever you choose to do, you will probably have to live with the emotional repercussions of that decision for the rest of your life.

If you are in the position of having to decide whether to have an invasive test such as amniocentesis which carries a slight risk of miscarriage, or if you are having to make the even harder decision about whether to end your pregnancy, your emotions are likely to be in turmoil. It's very hard to think clearly when you're so upset. Whilst bringing logic to bear might seem rather cold-hearted and extremely difficult, it is useful to have some strategy for trying to reach the decision that is best for you.

It may be helpful to write down the pros and cons of different courses of action so that you can literally 'see' what the issues are. Try making lists in the following way:

Decision A (e.g. to have an amniocentesis)

Decision B (e.g. not to have an amniocentesis)

What are the Benefits if I do this? (for me and my baby)
What are the Risks? (physical and emotional)
Are there any Alternatives?

If you can talk through the issues calmly with your partner or a friend using this kind of framework, the right decision might become clearer to you even if it's not easier to make.

Thinking Ahead

Since you are now reading this book, it's clear that you are already thinking ahead! It's very important when you are making decisions about antenatal tests to be able to do this. The shock of receiving bad news is infinitely harder for people who haven't thought ahead than for those who have discussed the tests beforehand, know what the different kinds of results mean and have considered what steps they would take if their baby appeared to have a problem. In the next chapters, you can read about other women's experiences of testing and the information given will help you consider all your options so that you can make the best decisions for you.

Key Points

- You don't *have* to have any antenatal tests at all.
- It's not true that you can only have tests if you agree to terminate your pregnancy should your baby prove to have Down's Syndrome or some other serious disabling condition.
- Get information about the tests from different sources – your GP, midwife, consultant, friends who have recently been pregnant, leaflets and books.
- Ask whether there is a midwife at your local hospital who specializes in counselling women and their families about antenatal testing.
- The important thing is to think ahead and make plans for what you will do if test results bring bad news. It's easier to cope if you know what your options are.

1

What the Tests Test For

What Do Antenatal Tests Tell You About Your Baby?

Most people associate antenatal testing with Down's Syndrome, the most common condition which the tests aim to detect. The tests also look for spina bifida and other rarer conditions which it's useful to know a little about so that you can understand what it would mean if your baby was born with one of them. There are literally hundreds of different genetic disorders which might be picked up by antenatal tests, and it can be impossible even for the most highly trained medical expert to know exactly what the implications of some of these might be. So you could be told that your baby's genetic make-up is different from that of most other babies but no-one can explain to you exactly what this might mean. However, such dilemmas are rare and this chapter concentrates on explaining what is involved in the conditions which are generally associated with antenatal testing.

Genetic Conditions

Down's Syndrome

Down's Syndrome is a *genetic* condition which means that from the moment of conception, the baby has Down's Syndrome; it's not a condition that develops while the baby is in the womb. Every cell in our body has 46 chromosomes which are arranged in 23 pairs. Each chromosome carries a huge amount of information in the form of *genes* and it is our genes which make each of us a unique individual. Instead of having just a pair of the number 21 chromosomes, people with Down's Syndrome have an extra chromosome. Doctors therefore describe their condition as *Tri*somy 21.

You have almost certainly met a person with Down's Syndrome or at least seen one. People with Down's Syndrome have a typical appearance – they are short in stature and thick-set; they have wide-set eyes, round faces and short necks. About 1,000 babies who have Down's Syndrome are born each year in the UK. The majority have problems with their heart and lungs and all have learning difficulties. By the time they reach adulthood, many people with Down's have the intellectual abilities of a child at junior school. They may be socially more skilled than a young child, however, and understand how to behave appropriately when mixing with other adults. Some decades ago, people with Down's had a very short life expectancy, but nowadays, may live until they are 50 or more.

If you want to find out more about Down's Syndrome and what it means to the people who have it and to their families, you could contact the Down's Syndrome Association. This book includes an account of the birth of a little girl with Down's Syndrome and of the family to which she belongs (see Chapter 8).

Edward's Syndrome

Whereas babies who have Down's Syndrome have an extra twenty-first chromosome, a baby who has Edward's Syndrome has an extra eighteenth chromosome. The baby's head is small and he or she has a flat forehead and a receding chin. Sadly, because babies who have Edward's Syndrome nearly always have problems with their heart, lungs and digestive organs, they are unable to live for long and the majority die during their first year of life.

Edward's Syndrome is not common. About one in every 5,000 babies has this condition.

Patau's Syndrome

This is another condition which is caused by an extra chromosome. A baby who has Patau's Syndrome has an extra thirteenth chromosome. The baby's face and limbs do not form normally and the heart, kidneys and brain may also be affected. Most children who have Patau's Syndrome live only for two or three years.

Turner's Syndrome

Only girl babies can have Turner's Syndrome. The condition is caused by a mistake in the chromosomes which control the sex of the baby. Normally, girls have two 'X' sex chromosomes whilst boys have an 'X' and a 'Y' sex chromosome. Babies who have Turner's Syndrome have just one 'X' chromosome. In appearance, they have short, thick necks and swollen feet and nipples that are spaced very widely apart. Their sexual organs don't develop properly. Women who have Turner's Syndrome are not able to have babies themselves but they are usually of normal intelligence and can lead normal lives as adults.

Cystic Fibrosis

Cystic fibrosis (CF) affects about one in 500 people. It is a genetic condition which is passed from one generation to the next. CF affects the lungs and digestive system. The lungs are normally kept moist by secretions which enable them to function properly, and our digestion is helped by secretions from the pancreas which break down the food we eat so that it can be absorbed into our bodies. Babies who have cystic fibrosis have very thick secretions in their lungs and digestive tract so that they are vulnerable to pneumonia and bronchitis and need dietary supplements, especially vitamins to ensure that they are properly nourished. The disease is often very serious and most people who have cystic fibrosis have a life expectancy of only 20 to 30 years.

Congenital Conditions

Spina Bifida

Spina bifida is a *congenital* condition. Babies with spina bifida have normal genes; the problem for them occurred after conception while they were growing in the womb. The way in which a baby develops in his mother's womb is an amazingly complex process. It's hardly surprising that sometimes not every part of the baby develops as it should. Perhaps what is really surprising is that 'mistakes' happen so rarely. People who have spina bifida have a gap in the bones of their spine so that the precious spinal cord which lies underneath is damaged. The spinal cord is responsible for carrying messages from all the nerves of the body to the brain so that we can move our limbs, feel sensations such as heat, cold and pain, know when we want to go to the toilet and so on.

You may know people who don't know they have spina bifida. In their case, the gap in the bones of the spine is so small that the cord underneath is not damaged and their nervous system works normally. This is called spina bifida occulta which means 'hidden' or 'closed' spina bifida. Some people with closed spina bifida do have problems with moving their limbs and with bladder and bowel control, but they are not seriously disabled by their condition. This kind of spina bifida *cannot* be detected by an antenatal blood test.

Babies born with more serious spina bifida may be paralysed in the lower part of their bodies so that they cannot move their legs. They will never learn to walk or to control their bladders or bowels when they grow older. Some babies who have spina bifida also have hydrocephalus. This means that they have a lot of fluid in their heads. Babies born with hydrocephalus can have surgery so that the excess fluid is shunted into their bloodstream, but even if a shunt is put in shortly after birth, it may be too late to prevent pressure on the brain causing damage which may result in learning difficulties later on.

The number of babies born with spina bifida varies across the United Kingdom. Some areas such as the Northeast, South Wales and Scotland have more babies with spina bifida than others so that whilst only 2 per 1,000 women in the south of the country might be pregnant with babies who have spina bifida, there are likely to be 6 in Scotland.

Today, about 30 per cent of babies born with spina bifida go to school although many of these children have very serious disabilities. 70 per cent of babies with spina bifida die in the first few years of their lives.

The Association for Spina Bifida and Hydrocephalus helps people with spina bifida and their carers. You can get more information by telephoning or writing to them. The address and phone number are given at the end of this book.

Anencephaly

Anencephaly is another congenital condition. The top part of the baby's skull does not develop properly and the brain may not grow at all. The majority of babies who are born with anencephaly are girls. None of these infants can survive; some live just for a few minutes or perhaps a few hours.

Gastroschisis and Exomphalos

Babies who have gastroschisis have a gap in the skin and muscle which form the wall of their abdomen so that some of their internal organs grow outside their bodies. Exomphalos is similar except that with this condition there is a lining over the bulge outside the abdomen and with gastroschisis there is no lining. Exomphalos and gastroschisis happen about once in every 5,000 births. They are conditions which are often spotted when the mother has an ultrasound scan and although there is no treatment for the baby until he is born, it's usually fairly easy to put the organs which are outside back inside and to sew up the hole in the abdominal wall. Gastroschisis is generally a one-off condition, but babies born with exomphalos sometimes have other problems as well.

Further Information and Support

Voluntary Organizations

There are many, many voluntary organizations which aim to help parents who have or might have a child with a physical or mental health problem. These organizations are largely run by parents who have disabled children themselves. Voluntary organizations have often put time and money into research and have gathered together a wealth of information and practical advice which they can offer to people who contact them as well as having a deep understanding of how parents feel in difficult situations. They are regularly asked for their advice by health professionals. If you discover that your unborn baby has a health problem, it's always a good idea to contact the relevant voluntary organization and speak to a parent who can tell you what the condition might mean for the child and for you as his parents. You will find yourself speaking to people who are not only extremely knowledgeable, but who also have the time to talk to you and are committed to helping people in your position. The volunteers who work for such organizations have generally received training in counselling and they will not be in any way judgemental or attempt to persuade you into a particular decision.

Antenatal Tests for the Mother

Pregnancy tests monitor not only your baby's health but also your own. Whilst many of the tests which women have during pregnancy are routine, some are highly specialized and available only if you are considered at high risk of having a condition which may affect your baby's (and your own) well-being. Remember that the decision about whether to go ahead with any particular test is always yours.

Blood Tests

Women get used to having blood taken during pregnancy; it becomes a routine procedure for most people unless you have a needle phobia when it's far from routine and extremely traumatic. If you're frightened of needles, find out at which antenatal appointments your midwife will need to take blood and make sure you have your partner or a friend with you.

When you see your midwife or GP in order to have your pregnancy confirmed and to talk about where you want your baby to be born, you will be asked to give a blood sample. This will be tested for:

- blood group: (A, B, AB or O)
- antibodies: (substances in your blood which could pass to your baby and cause her to bleed after she is born)
- Rhesus factor: (positive or negative)
- haemoglobin level: (to see whether you are anaemic)
- platelet level: (platelets are blood cells which control clotting)
- white cell level: (white blood cells fight off infection)
- rubella status: (to see if you are immune to rubella [German measles])
- hepatitis B
- syphilis

Blood Group and Antibodies

Your blood group is checked so that if you lose a lot of blood when you give birth to your baby, there will be no delay in giving you the right transfusion. If you have religious objections to blood transfusions, you need to state this clearly and ensure that your doctor or midwife writes in your notes that you will not accept a transfusion. Your blood is also checked for antibodies to see if there is any incompatibility between your blood and your baby's. The most common incompatibility is associated with the Rhesus Factor.

Rhesus Factor

Being Rhesus negative is only a problem if your baby is Rhesus positive but as there's no easy way of knowing what your baby's blood type is, it's considered best to keep a close eye on every pregnant woman who is Rhesus negative. During pregnancy, a few of your baby's red blood cells will get into your circulation. If you do not have the Rhesus factor in your blood (i.e. you are Rhesus negative) but your baby does (i.e. is Rhesus positive) your body will recognize that the baby's blood cells are different from yours and will therefore consider them dangerous. It will start to make antibodies to attack the foreign cells and eventually, these antibodies cross the placenta and start to destroy your baby's red blood cells.

Babies who are born with Rhesus disease are very poorly indeed and may need many blood transfusions. They are anaemic and jaundiced and sometimes have serious liver damage.

However, Rhesus disease in this country is largely a thing of the past. If you are pregnant for the first time, your body will not manufacture enough antibodies to affect your baby during this pregnancy. Problems might arise during your next pregnancy if you have another Rhesus positive baby, because your body will already have a system in place for producing antibodies to your baby's blood cells. In order to prevent a subsequent pregnancy running into problems, you will be offered an injection of Anti-D after your first baby is born to ensure that your next pregnancy is not at risk. The injection destroys any antibodies which your body has already manufactured.

Haemoglobin

It's normal to be slightly anaemic during pregnancy because your blood volume increases substantially but you still have the same number of red blood cells. So you have fewer red blood cells in 20 ml of blood than a non-pregnant woman has in the same amount of blood. Some women, however, are truly anaemic during pregnancy either because they have poor health or a poor diet or because their pregnancy is making such heavy demands on their bodies. These women need extra iron to help them make more red blood cells.

Platelets and White Cells

Platelets are blood cells which help your blood to clot when you have an injury, either internal or external. During pregnancy, your platelet levels may drop a little and this is normal, but if they drop too far, you may be at risk of a haemorrhaging when you give birth. If your midwife and doctor know that your platelet count is low, they will be able to give you extra attention during your labour.

The number of white blood cells in your blood indicates whether you have an infection, although not what kind of infection it might be. If your white cell count is very high, your doctor will want to talk to you about your health and find out whether there is a problem which could be treated.

Rubella

There has been a lot of health education in recent years about the importance of pregnant women avoiding contact with people who have rubella (which used to be called German measles). If a woman catches rubella in the first four months of pregnancy, her baby may be infected by the virus because it crosses the placenta. This is extremely serious. The baby may be born blind or deaf. He may have heart problems and severe learning difficulties.

The blood which is taken at your booking visit is tested to see whether you are immune to rubella. Most women are because they've had the illness (even if it wasn't diagnosed) when they were small. If you are not immune to rubella, you will be advised to keep away from anyone – and especially children – who have or may have the infection.

If your blood test shows that you have recently had rubella and you are still in the early months of pregnancy, you will be offered a termination because it is very likely that your baby will be seriously damaged by the virus. The choice is always yours as to whether you want to end your pregnancy or continue with it.

Hepatitis B

In many clinics, pregnant women are routinely tested for hepatitis B which is an extremely common virus. Millions of people the world over are carriers which means that they have no obvious symptoms of the disease although they are infected with the virus. Some people are especially at risk of hepatitis B infection such as health professionals and laboratory workers who work with blood or blood products. People who inject illegal drugs may become infected through sharing needles with other addicts. Sometimes people who have had a tattoo develop hepatitis B because the needles which were used to tattoo them were dirty. You may be at risk of hepatitis B if you have recently visited a country where the disease is very common.

The blood test for hepatitis B tells you whether you have the virus and whether it is infectious. If it is, there is a risk that your baby will be born with hepatitis B. He will need early treatment with vaccine to protect him from developing chronic liver disease.

Syphilis

Most women are surprised to find that their blood is being tested for syphilis which is a rare disease in this country. However, if the mother does have syphilis, the effects on her baby are likely to be very serious indeed. Babies who are born with syphilis have a large spleen and liver; they are anaemic and jaundiced and may have learning difficulties.

If your blood test shows that you have syphilis, you will be offered treatment with antibiotics. The antibiotics cross the placenta to your baby so that he or she is treated at the same time. A long course of antibiotics may be necessary and you will have your blood tested at regular intervals to assess how effective the antibiotics are being.

Special Tests

Testing for Sickle-Cell Disease

If you are of African, Caribbean, Mediterranean, Middle Eastern or Indian origin, you will be asked if the blood sample taken at your booking visit can be tested for sickle-cell.

Sickle-cell disease is a genetic condition which programmes the bone marrow to manufacture sickle-shaped red blood cells rather than the normal spherical ones. The reason why this genetic mutation occurred in some parts of the world is because sickle-shaped red blood cells protect people from malaria which is a serious hazard in many countries. However, the sickle-shaped cells themselves cause problems in that they can block blood vessels giving rise to a sickle-cell crisis which is extremely painful and may be life-threatening.

If you have sickle-cell disease, your pregnancy could be a difficult one. The circulation of blood through the placenta may become blocked in places so that your baby receives less oxygen and food. You may go into labour early and your baby might be quite small because he or she hasn't grown very well in the womb.

You have to have two sickle-cell genes (pieces of genetic information) in order to have sickle-cell disease. A baby whose mother and father both have sickle-cell disease will also have sickle-cell disease. Many people, however, only have one sickle-cell gene and they are then said to have sickle-cell *trait*. Very often, men and women with sickle-cell trait have no symptoms, although they may have a tendency to be anaemic. A baby born to a man and woman who both have sickle-cell trait has a one in four chance of having sickle-cell disease.

The pattern is different if only one parent has sickle-cell trait. Statistically half of the babies born to this couple will have normal blood and half will have sickle-cell trait. Another way of putting this is to say that each baby has a 50/50 chance of having normal blood or of having sickle-cell trait.

If one parent has sickle-cell disease and the other parent doesn't, then all the babies born to this couple will have sickle-cell trait although none will have sickle-cell disease.

If you already know that you have sickle-cell disease or if a blood test shows that you have sickle-cell trait, your partner will be asked to have a blood test as well. Don't worry if this is not possible; it's simply helpful in estimating the likelihood of your baby having sickle-cell disease. If there is a strong possibility that your baby will have sickle-cell disease, you can talk to your consultant about the best place for you to give birth to ensure that he can receive immediate expert attention.

Testing for Thalassaemia

If you are of Mediterranean, Middle Eastern or South East Asian origin, you will be offered a blood test for thalassaemia.

Like sickle-cell disease, thalassaemia is a genetic condition and in order to have the disease, you have to have two identical pieces of genetic information in each body cell. If you have only one gene for thalassaemia, you have thalassaemia *trait* which may well cause you no problems at all but could become a problem for your baby if your partner also has thalassaemia trait. So if a blood test shows that you have the trait, your partner will also be asked to have a blood test so that your baby's risk of being affected by thalassaemia can be estimated. The pattern of inheritance is the same as for sickle-cell disease (see above).

If a baby is born with what is called thalassaemia major – that is she received a thalassaemia gene from both parents – she may be so ill that she dies quite soon after birth. Because her red blood cells are not formed properly, they are broken down by her body very quickly and she becomes seriously anaemic. This puts a tremendous strain on her heart. Some babies do survive but they need regular blood transfusions throughout their lives and this is a huge challenge for both the person with thalassaemia and for her carers.

Testing for Tay-Sachs Disease

This is a genetic disease which can only be passed on to a baby if both parents are carriers of the disease. It is a very serious condition which affects the baby's brain from when he or she is about six months old. Babies with Tay-Sachs live for only three or four years.

Although quite a few people in the general population are carriers of Tay-Sachs, people who are Ashkenazi Jews are particularly likely to be carriers. As many as 1 person in every 25 Ashkenazi Jews is a carrier. Carriers are perfectly healthy.

If you or your partner is Jewish, you will probably be offered a blood test when you first see your doctor or midwife to find out whether you are a carrier. If you are, your partner will also be asked to give some blood for testing. Should you both prove to be carriers, you will then need to decide whether you want to have chorionic villus sampling or amniocentesis to find out whether your baby has Tay-Sachs disease. There is a one in four chance that this will be the case.

Remember that if you feel that under no circumstances would you choose to terminate your pregnancy, you can refuse to have either the blood test or the diagnostic tests. Nobody should put you under any pressure to accept testing.

Testing for Toxoplasmosis

Toxoplasmosis is an infection which is caught by eating anything infected with the parasite *Toxoplasma gondii*. The parasite can be found in rare or raw meat, cat mess, soil contaminated by cat mess, and unpasteurized goat's milk. Many people will have toxoplasmosis in their lives and never know as the mild flu-like symptoms often go unnoticed.

Toxoplasmosis is dangerous to babies if a woman catches the infection for the first time just before she conceives or in the early part of her pregnancy. If this is the case there is a chance that the baby will become infected, with a risk of brain damage, eye damage, and damage to other organs. The risk of the baby becoming infected is 40 per cent overall, but lower in early pregnancy and higher in later pregnancy. The damage that can be caused is less severe later in pregnancy, so most babies born with toxoplasmosis have some degree of eye damage but will not have the more severe symptoms (such as hydrocephalus).

It is thought that 50–60 babies a year are born with severe congenital toxoplasmosis. In this country pregnant women are not routinely screened for toxoplasmosis as it is considered too expensive – in any case, it would cause too much unnecessary anxiety, as the vast majority of women aren't at risk.

If you are worried about toxoplasmosis, you need to talk to your midwife or doctor about having a blood test. A positive blood test means that you have had toxoplasmosis at some time in your life. A positive result also means it is likely you have an immunity which will protect you and your baby. However, further specialized blood tests must be done at a Toxoplasma Reference Unit: these tests will tell you whether or not the infection was recent enough to present a risk to your baby. If your baby is at risk then treatment with an antibiotic called spiramycin can reduce the chances of the baby becoming infected by 50–60 per cent.

The best way to deal with toxoplasmosis before and during pregnancy is to avoid getting it in the first place.

Toxoplasmosis: Minimizing the Risk

- ❑ Don't eat raw or undercooked meat, and wash your hands and utensils after preparing raw meat.
- ❑ Wear gloves for gardening, and always wash your hands afterwards.
- ❑ Wash fruit and vegetables thoroughly to remove all traces of soil.
- ❑ Take care when changing cat litter trays. Clear out faeces daily, wear gloves, and wash your hands afterwards.
- ❑ Don't drink unpasteurized milk, goat's milk, or goat's milk products.
- ❑ If you work on a farm, avoid helping with lambing while you are pregnant.

Testing for Cystic Fibrosis

Lots of white people (about 1 in 25) are carriers of a single cystic fibrosis gene without knowing it because being a carrier means that you have no symptoms of the disease. However, if a man and a woman who are both CF carriers have a baby, the baby has a one in four chance of having the disease. African Caribbean people and Asian people are much less likely than white people to be carriers of cystic fibrosis. Ashkenazi Jews are much more likely to be carriers of one particular kind of cystic fibrosis.

The diagram below shows how people who are carriers of the

cystic fibrosis gene may pass the disease on to their baby. Each cell of the parents' bodies has one gene for cystic fibrosis matched with one normal gene (genes are always arranged in pairs). Because at conception, the mother and father both give one gene to their baby, there is a 50 per cent chance that their baby will be a carrier of cystic fibrosis; there is a 25 per cent chance that their baby will have two normal genes, and there is a 25 per cent chance that their baby will have cystic fibrosis.

❑ When both parents are CF carriers:

Mother	Father	Baby	Outcome
CF gene + normal gene	CF gene + normal gene	CF gene + normal gene	this baby is a carrier of cystic fibrosis but doesn't have any symptoms (like his/her parents)
CF gene + normal gene	CF gene + normal gene	normal gene + normal gene	this baby doesn't have cystic fibrosis and isn't a carrier
CF gene + normal gene	CF gene + normal gene	CF gene + CF gene	this baby has cystic fibrosis

If either you or your partner has a close relative with cystic fibrosis, you might want to find out whether you yourselves are carriers of the CF gene so that you know whether your baby is at risk. Where there is a family history of cystic fibrosis, you will probably be asked by your midwife or doctor if you would like to have a carrier test. If you are worried about cystic fibrosis but do not come from a family where there is someone affected by the disease, you will probably have to have the test done privately and pay for it yourself. If you decide to do this, it's a good idea to let your GP know so that he or she can be contacted by the screening service with the results.

The test involves both you and your partner providing a mouthwash sample. Your sample will be tested first and if you are a carrier of cystic fibrosis, your partner's sample will also be tested. If you are not a carrier, your partner's sample will not be tested because you both have to be carriers for there to be a risk of your baby having CF. You should receive a result within 10 days of posting your samples to the screening service if you are having the test done privately, or within 10 days of your doctor sending the samples to the laboratory.

The result will tell you whether you are at high risk of having a baby with cystic fibrosis or at low risk. The mouthwash test cannot tell you for certain whether your baby has cystic fibrosis. If you are at low risk, you could still have a baby with cystic fibrosis because the CF gene has many different forms and, at the moment, the test can only detect some of these. So you and your partner could both be carriers of a rare form of CF which the test cannot detect. Remember that even if both you and your partner are found to be carriers of cystic fibrosis, your baby still has a three in four chance of not being affected by the disease.

If you get a 'high risk' result, you can choose to have further tests such as chorionic villus sampling or amniocentesis to find out for certain whether your baby has cystic fibrosis. Before making a decision, ask to speak to the hospital's Genetic Counsellor if there is one, or a doctor or midwife who can tell you about cystic fibrosis and consider your risk with you. If you are not happy with the counselling you receive, or want to talk to parents of children with CF, you can contact the Cystic Fibrosis Trust. (see address list at end of book)

Testing for HIV/AIDS

In some clinics, every pregnant woman's blood is tested to see whether she has HIV antibodies. However, this is not a 'named test' which means that the results can't be traced back to the individual woman who gave the blood. It's simply a means of collecting data to see how fast HIV is spreading. Even if your blood is only going to be tested anonymously, your midwife should ask your permission.

You might want to consider having a *named* HIV test during your pregnancy. Perhaps you feel that you are at risk because you have had intercourse with a partner whom you know or suspect is positive, or because you have shared needles to inject drugs or because your life-style puts you at risk of HIV. If you are of African origin, or have lived in Africa recently, you may find that your midwife or doctor tries quite hard to persuade you to have an HIV test because it is known that HIV is very common in some African countries.

The decision about whether to have a named test is certainly not an easy one. To find out that you are positive feels like receiving a death sentence because although many people with HIV live a normal, healthy life for a large number of years, there are still no drugs available to prevent HIV eventually developing into AIDS and there is still no cure for AIDS. You may decide that you and those around you would find it impossible to cope with knowing that you are HIV positive. You may fear that your partner will leave you if he finds out you are positive or that he will react violently. You may also be frightened that your baby will be taken away from you if you are known to be positive although this alone is never a reason for taking a baby into care. You are not putting your doctor and midwife at risk if you decide not to find out whether you are positive, because it is their responsibility to bear in mind that any woman for whom they are caring could have HIV and to take the proper precautions to protect themselves at all times.

On the other hand, you may feel that pregnancy is the right time for you to find out whether you are positive so that you can make plans to protect both your own health and your baby's. If you know that you are positive, you can make choices about:

- whether to have treatment with anti-viral drugs during pregnancy (although these drugs are still being tested and not every clinic will offer them)
- where to have your baby so that you can both receive the best treatment (babies born to positive women who are well are not more likely to be premature or underweight, but the more ill the mother is with HIV, the more likely the baby is to be poorly)
- how your baby should be born (caesarean birth *may* reduce the chances of a baby becoming positive)
- how to feed your baby (the World Health Organization recommends that positive women should bottle-feed their babies if they live in countries where there is a clean water supply and formula milk is easily available)
- who will look after your baby if you become ill.

There is about a one in seven chance that the baby of a woman who is HIV positive will also have HIV although it's generally not possible to be sure about the baby until she is about 18 months old. This is because all babies born to mothers with HIV have HIV antibodies in their blood which have passed to them across the placenta. Until the baby's immune system has developed, it's not possible to say whether she is manufacturing her own antibodies to her own HIV infection. Some clinics offer tests which look for the HIV virus itself rather than for antibodies to the virus and this makes it possible to find out whether the baby is positive when she is about three months old.

If you are thinking about having an HIV test, you need to ask your midwife whether there is a trained counsellor at the hospital who can talk to you. If there isn't and she herself is not able to discuss the issues fully with you, you can ring The Terrence Higgins Trust or Positively Women which offer professional counselling and support to people who have or suspect they may have HIV. Positively Women is based in London but is in the process of setting up satellite centres in other cities and very often, someone from the organization will come to see you in person if you need to talk (see address list at end of book).

Urine Testing

At each clinic visit, you will be asked to give a sample of urine. If you are the kind of person who finds it impossible to go to the toilet when specifically requested to do so, ask your midwife for a specimen pot to take home and fill it just before you come for your next antenatal check. This will avoid the embarrassment of not being able to produce a sample!

Pre-eclampsia

Your urine is tested principally for two things – sugar and protein. The tests can be carried out quickly by your midwife either in the antenatal clinic or at home. If you have protein in your urine, it may be a sign of a condition called pre-eclampsia. Nobody is quite sure what causes pre-eclampsia but its effect is to cause your blood pressure to become dangerously high so that the placenta stops functioning properly and your baby is starved of oxygen and food. You yourself might develop serious problems with your liver and kidneys and with clots in your blood.

The signs of pre-eclampsia are:

- blood pressure getting higher during the second half of pregnancy
- protein in the urine
- swelling of the face, hands, ankles and feet although such swelling is also common in women who do *not* have pre-eclampsia.

Many women find that their ankles swell when they are heavily pregnant, or that their rings become tight because of swelling in their hands. This is simply because the size of the baby inside makes blood circulation less efficient. The swelling has nothing to do with pre-eclampsia; it's just an ordinary side-effect of being pregnant. For this reason your midwife won't consider that you have pre-eclampsia if you have no other symptoms apart from swelling. Having raised blood-pressure or protein in your urine are much more important and reliable symptoms.

Occasionally, pre-eclampsia comes 'out of the blue' even though the tests you have had at your antenatal appointments have been normal. You will know that something is wrong if you experience any of the following:

- visual disturbances such as spots before your eyes
- pain in the upper half of your tummy
- sickness

If you have any of these symptoms and you know that they are not due to a migraine or to eating something which has disagreed with you, you should ring your midwife, GP or the hospital where you are booked to give birth (if you are not having a home birth) and ask for advice.

Pregnancy Diabetes

Your urine is also tested for sugar. This is because some women develop diabetes during pregnancy which means that you have too much sugar in your blood because your pancreas is not producing enough insulin to turn the sugar into stored energy. Diabetes makes you feel thirsty and sluggish and it's not good for your baby who may grow very big as a result of all the sugar coming across the placenta.

If you have a lot of sugar in your urine, your midwife or doctor will want to do a glucose tolerance test (GTT). You will be asked to have nothing to eat from midnight and to come to the antenatal clinic first thing in the morning to have your blood taken. This first sample of blood gives a baseline reading for the level of sugar in your blood when you've had nothing to eat for a long time. Next, you will be asked to swallow 75 g of glucose mixture which you will probably find disgustingly sweet! After an hour, another sample of blood will be taken. Further samples are taken after two hours and after three. If you find having your blood taken very traumatic, bring your partner or a friend with you so that you have someone to hold your hand and encourage you.

By comparing the three samples of blood taken after you had the glucose drink with the sample taken before, your doctor can tell whether your body is producing enough insulin to keep your blood sugar at the right level. If there seems to be a problem, you will be referred to a specialist in diabetes who will discuss your diet with you and how to control your blood sugar level by taking tablets or having injections of insulin.

Many women who are diagnosed with pregnancy diabetes do not go on being diabetic after their babies are born. However, they may be more at risk of developing diabetes in later life than women who haven't had pregnancy diabetes.

What Your Blood Is Tested for

At 'Booking' (12 weeks of pregnancy)

- ❑ blood group
- ❑ Rhesus factor
- ❑ haemoglobin level
- ❑ antibodies, platelets and white cells
- ❑ syphilis
- ❑ rubella immunity
- ❑ hepatitis B

Perhaps:

- ❑ sickle–cell disease
- ❑ thalassaemia
- ❑ HIV

At 28 Weeks

- ❑ haemoglobin levels
- ❑ Rhesus antibodies if you are Rhesus negative

At 32 weeks

- ❑ Rhesus antibodies if you are Rhesus negative

At 36 weeks

- ❑ haemoglobin level
- ❑ Rhesus antibodies if you are Rhesus negative

At 40 weeks

- ❑ Rhesus antibodies if you are Rhesus negative

3

Blood Tests

Screening Tests and Diagnostic Tests

Before you read this chapter, it's important to remind yourself of the difference between a screening test and a diagnostic test.

SCREENING TEST
A screening test tells you what your *risk* is of having a baby with Down's Syndrome or spina bifida

DIAGNOSTIC TEST
A diagnostic test tells you for certain whether your baby has Down's Syndrome or spina bifida (or some other serious condition)

Being Certain of Your Dates

Blood tests to screen for Down's Syndrome and spina bifida are only useful if you know for certain how many weeks pregnant you are. Some women are sure of the date when they conceived and many are sure of the first day of their last period which enables the midwife to make a fairly good estimate of when they are due to have their babies. If you are not sure how many weeks pregnant you are when you first see your GP or midwife (and even if you are) you will probably be offered an ultrasound scan to assess what stage your pregnancy is at. Scans which are carried out in the first thirteen weeks of pregnancy are very accurate in determining when the baby is due.

Blood tests to check your baby are carried out when you are between 16 and 18 weeks pregnant. Your blood may be tested for one, two or three different substances or 'markers' depending on how sophisticated the test is which your hospital provides. Sometimes, a fourth marker is added.

Markers

+ alphafeto protein (AFP)
+ human chorionic gonadotrophin (HCG)
+ unconjugated estriols
+ inhibin-A or neutrophil alkaline phosphatase

Most women nowadays have a 'double' or 'triple' test which means that two or three markers are being looked at, although you may hear your blood test described simply as the AFP test and presume that it is just the level of alphafeto protein which is being measured.

If you are unsure how many markers your hospital is using, ask for more information.

Understanding the Results of Your Blood Test

If your blood test shows that your risk of being pregnant with a baby who has Down's Syndrome is less than 1 in 250, your result will be described as **SCREEN NEGATIVE**.

*This does not mean that you definitely **aren't** pregnant with a baby who has Down's Syndrome.*

It only means that it's very unlikely that your baby has Down's Syndrome.

If your blood test shows that your risk of being pregnant with a baby who has Down's Syndrome is more than 1 in 250, your result will be described as **SCREEN POSITIVE**.

*This does not mean that you definitely **are** pregnant with a baby who has Down's Syndrome.*

In fact, the likelihood of your baby having Down's Syndrome is still very low.

Testing for Down's Syndrome

When your blood is tested to see whether you might be carrying a baby who has Down's Syndrome, the level of alphafeto protein (AFP) will be measured and also the level of human chorionic gonadotrophin (HCG). A third and fourth marker may also be measured. These markers can also be used to estimate your risk of carrying a baby who has Edward's Syndrome although this condition is much more rare than Down's Syndrome, and some other genetic conditions which are even rarer. The reason why several markers are used is because AFP testing alone for Down's Syndrome is not very reliable and the more markers that are used, the more reliable the results of the screening test become. However, it's important to remember that blood tests for Down's Syndrome are screening tests and therefore will identify some babies as being at risk who do not have Down's Syndrome and will miss some who do.

Here's an example to help explain why so many Down's Syndrome babies are 'missed' despite widespread antenatal testing:

If you take a group of 10,000 pregnant women and offer them all a triple test,

2,500 women will refuse the test because they wouldn't consider a termination even if their baby was found to have Down's Syndrome.

Amongst these 2,500 pregnant women, there will be about 4 who are carrying Down's Syndrome babies.

– 4 MISSED –

Of the remaining 7,500 women who accept the triple test, there will be about 7 whose test results are *screen negative* but who *are* carrying babies with Down's Syndrome.

– 7 MISSED –

Of the 375 women who are screen positive with the triple test, 95 decide against having an amniocentesis because the miscarriage risk is not acceptable to them. Amongst these 95 women, 1 or 2 will be carrying a baby who has Down's Syndrome.

– 1 or 2 MISSED –

Of the remaining 280 who choose to have an amniocentesis, about 5 are found to be pregnant with babies who have Down's Syndrome.

TOTALS

- 14 BABIES WITH DOWN'S SYNDROME MISSED -
- 5 BABIES WITH DOWN'S SYNDROME IDENTIFIED -
(based on *Modern Midwife*, June 1995)

As tests become more highly developed, the accuracy improves, but screening tests by definition do not give a straight yes/no answer.

Taking Your Age into Account

The chances that you are carrying a baby who has Down's Syndrome increase with age. A very young mother has only a tiny chance of having a baby with Down's Syndrome, and a mother who is over 40 has quite a high chance.

Age of the Mother and Risk of Down's Syndrome

Mother's Age	Chance of Down's
under 25 years	1:1,500
25 years	1:1,350
30 years	1:910
35 years	1:380
40 years	1:110
45 years	1:30
50 years	1:6

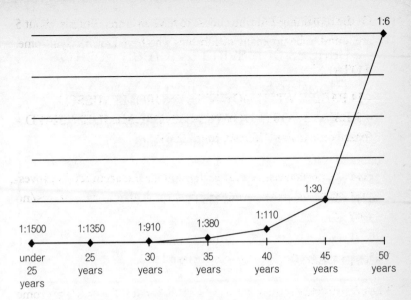

RISK OF DOWN'S SYNDROME ACCORDING TO MOTHER'S AGE

If you have an alphafeto protein test or the double or triple test, your age will be taken into account when your risk of having a baby with Down's Syndrome is estimated. So if your risk according to the levels of AFP and HCG in your blood is very low and your age-related risk is very low, your overall risk will be very low indeed. If your age-related risk is very high, it is likely that your blood will screen positive whatever the levels of AFP and HCG because your age will strongly influence the final calculation. This is why many women who are 40 years or over will screen positive when they have a blood test.

Chances of Having a Screen Positive
Blood Test According to Your Age

Mother's Age	Chances of Having a Screen Positive Result
under 25 years	1 in 40
25–29 years	1 in 30
30–34 years	1 in 15
35–39 years	1 in 5
40–44 years	1 in 3
45 years and over	more than 1 in 2

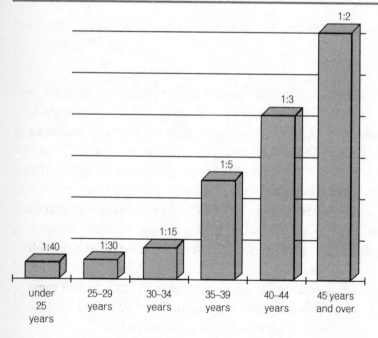

RISK OF SCREEN POSITIVE RESULT ACCORDING TO MOTHER'S AGE

Because of this, older women may decide not to have a blood test and to opt straightaway for amniocentesis. There doesn't seem much point in having a test which is almost bound to be positive and then making another appointment to have an amniocentesis. Many hospitals routinely offer amniocentesis to all women over the age of 35. The result is that far fewer babies who have Down's Syndrome are born to women in this age group than to younger women because older women are more likely to find out that they are pregnant with a Down's Syndrome baby and many make the choice to end their pregnancies.

There are a number of factors besides your age which may affect the result of your blood test.

Reasons Why Your Blood Test Might Not Be Accurate

1 A woman who is very overweight may have lower levels of AFP and HCG than a woman of normal weight. Women who are underweight tend to have higher levels.
2 African-Caribbean women often have higher levels of AFP and HCG than white women.
3 Women who are pregnant with twins will have higher levels of AFP and HCG.
4 Women who have diabetes and need to inject themselves with insulin to control the disease tend to have lower levels of AFP.
5 Blood test results can be inaccurate if you have had some recent bleeding from the vagina. The test should be done again a week after the bleeding has stopped.

To a certain extent, it is possible to take these factors into account when assessing a woman's risk of carrying a baby who has Down's Syndrome, but the business of risk assessment is a very tricky one and it's not difficult to see why blood tests are relatively unreliable.

The more accurate the dating of the pregnancy, the more accurate the blood test will be. Lee had the triple test and was told that she was screen positive:

'It turned out that the result of the triple test was false because it had been done too early. When I had a scan prior to having an amniocentesis, the size of the baby confirmed that the blood test must have been invalid. I didn't have the amniocentesis. I had a second triple test which came back negative.'

Lee

If you think that you are not as pregnant as the hospital says, ask to have another blood test when *you* think it is the right time. Some women, like Nageena, know when their baby was conceived:

'I was able to give the hospital my date of conception but they refused to accept this and gave me an early scan to date the baby. I was told it was crucial that the blood tests were done in week 16, otherwise they would not be accurate. However, the scan dates did not match my own. I was concerned that the tests would be done at the wrong time, but was simply told that the scan was very accurate and I had got my dates wrong.'

Nageena

If you know the date your baby was conceived, no test in the world can give better information than you can!

Twins

If you are pregnant with twin babies, you can't find out from a blood test whether one or both or neither of your babies has Down's Syndrome because the results of one blood test can't be applied to two babies. It's harder to check twins for Down's Syndrome than a single baby because the doctor has to be able to look at each baby separately. Your options are to have the nuchal translucency test very early in your pregnancy, or to have an amniocentesis later on. For more details, see the chapters about these tests.

Getting the Results of Your Blood Test

Unfortunately, if your blood test is screen negative, which means that you have a very low risk of being pregnant with a baby who has Down's Syndrome, you probably won't be told the result at all. Many women consider this extremely unsatisfactory and wish that they could receive a short letter through the post to tell them that they are at low risk. It's a good idea to find out from the hospital at what point you can assume that your result is screen negative because you have heard nothing. Otherwise, you might find yourself suffering considerable anxiety.

> 'Although I initially welcomed the blood tests as a check on the baby's progress, I ultimately felt they caused more anxiety than if there had been no testing. The hospital I attended had a policy of not giving test results to everyone, but only contacting women with problems. I had to ask my community midwife to find out for me how long test results took to come through and hence how quickly I would be contacted if needed.'

> *Sharon*

If Your Result is Screen Positive

It's important to remind yourself again and again that a screen positive result does not mean that your baby definitely has Down's Syndrome. Sometimes your risk is presented to you in such a way that it sounds as though it must be bad news but there are always two ways of considering a risk factor:

> 'Not until the amniocentesis itself was I told that 1 in 89 odds meant that I was far more likely to be one of the 88! Until then, all the statistics had been given to me from the negative viewpoint.'

Marisa

If your result is screen positive, you will have to think about what you want to do next. Hospitals vary in the amount of help they give to women who are having to make difficult decisions about testing. Jane represents one extreme of hospital care:

> 'My consultant was extremely sensitive and supportive and offered to do the amniocentesis there and then or at a later date and gave us time to discuss the pros and cons. My husband and I had discussed such an event and had no hesitation in having the amniocentesis.'

Jane

and Shona, the other:

> 'I phoned many times with specific questions about things I didn't understand (around "high risk" and amniocentesis)

but I was fobbed off with comments like "this is quite common" and "don't worry." I was at my wits' end and finally made an appointment to see my consultant. He answered my questions but made me feel I was making something out of nothing.'

Shona

Your options include:

1 To do nothing: accepting that even a risk of 1 in 40, for example, still means that your baby is far more likely to be healthy than to have Down's Syndrome.
2 Amniocentesis: this will tell you for definite whether your baby has Down's Syndrome, but the procedure does carry a small risk of miscarriage and you will probably have to wait about three weeks for the results (see chapter on amniocentesis).
3 High resolution ultrasound scan: a skilled sonographer using a good scanning machine might be able to spot heart problems or webbing of your baby's neck which often go with Down's Syndrome. Or the sonographer might find nothing at all out of the ordinary which would be reassuring for you.

If Your Result is Screen Negative

Having read this book so far, you will not be one of the women who believes that a screen negative result proves that her baby is all right. A screen negative result is very reassuring, but you still have to accept that there is a risk, however small, that your baby will have Down's Syndrome.

Your options from this point on are:

1 To have no further tests and enjoy the rest of your pregnancy!
2 To have an ultrasound scan in the middle of your pregnancy so that you get further reassurance about the health of your baby.
3 To have an amniocentesis if you are still very anxious and are prepared to accept the small risk that you may miscarry your baby following the procedure.

'I saw my GP at 16 weeks so that he could take some blood for the AFP test. He said to me quite sternly that if a woman would on no account undergo a "therapeutic termination" should all the tests prove that the baby was disabled, then there was no point in him doing the tests.

'This lecture, coupled with my natural anxiety about what the test might show, made waiting for the result practically unbearable. At no point was it off my mind. From the day of the test, I found myself unable to talk about the baby or think of it as ever being likely to be born.

'After ten days, I was contacted by a hospital midwife who told me that I was 1 in 90 for Down's Syndrome. I made an immediate decision with her to have an amniocentesis which was followed by a further agonizing wait – worse than the first one. The results came back clear. It seemed like half my pregnancy had been used up in waiting and agonizing.

'My main grouse is that the AFP test is so inaccurate leading to alarm, anxiety and stress but I am glad testing is available, however rocky the road.'

Jess

Alphafeto Protein Testing for Spina Bifida

AFP testing has been used for quite a long time to screen babies for spina bifida. If the level of AFP in the mother's blood is very high, this may indicate that her baby has open spina bifida (the most serious kind) or anencephaly. More recently, it was noticed that women who are pregnant with Down's Syndrome babies tend to have low levels of AFP and so the test is now used to screen for Down's Syndrome as well.

Unfortunately, there is not a clear cut-off point for the AFP test which enables a doctor or midwife to say, 'Yes, this baby definitely has spina bifida' because the range of abnormal results overlaps with the range of normal results. However, if your AFP level is very high (in technical terms: more than 2.5 multiples of the median) there is about an 80 per cent likelihood that your baby has spina bifida or anencephaly.

You need to remember, though, that even a very high level of AFP does *not* definitely mean that your baby has spina bifida. There is still a margin of error and some women who screen positive for spina bifida with the AFP test will be carrying normal babies.

If your AFP blood test puts you at high risk, you will be invited to have another test to confirm the result. This is likely to be a high resolution ultrasound scan which you may be able to have at your own hospital if the equipment there is very up-to-date. Or you may be referred to a Regional Referral Unit with a better scanner. The high quality of the scan you will receive will not only enable your sonographer to check carefully that your baby's spine is properly formed but also to examine closely many of his other organs, including his heart, digestive tract and brain. You will probably be able to see the different parts of your baby very clearly - perhaps a positive spin-off to your referral. If at all possible, take your partner or a friend with you when you go for your detailed scan so that you can share the outcome together.

Mandy was 25 years old when she became pregnant. She chose to receive most of her antenatal care from her GP who explained to her about the AFP screening test which she decided to have.

The test was done when Mandy was 16 weeks pregnant and eight days later, her GP received a phone call from the laboratory to say that the AFP level was very high. The GP telephoned Mandy to tell her the result and invited her to come into the surgery the next morning so that they could discuss what to do next.

After a sleepless night, Mandy saw her GP at 9 o'clock the following morning. Together, they decided to arrange for Mandy to have an ultrasound scan at the large maternity hospital in the nearby city.

Mandy's detailed scan showed that her baby's spine and brain were properly formed. The hospital doctors decided to keep an eye on Mandy's pregnancy, partly because she was so anxious as a result of the tests. Mandy had a series of scans during the rest of her pregnancy to make sure that her baby was growing properly.

At 38 weeks, she gave birth to a healthy boy, weighing eight and a half pounds.

Mandy

Flow Chart for Blood Tests

ASK YOURSELF

> Shall I have a blood test?
> What will I do if the result is screen positive?

Refuse test   Accept AFP/Double/Triple test

Result: screen negative   Result: screen positive

ASK YOURSELF

> Do I want any more
> tests?
> Which tests?
> What will I do if the
> result is positive?

> Do I want any more
> tests?
> Which tests?
> What will I do if the
> result is positive?

No more tests   More tests   No more tests   More tests

ultrasound
amniocentesis

another blood test
amniocentesis
ultrasound

Blood Tests

Screening/Diagnostic	Screening
When Carried Out	16–18 weeks of pregnancy
Availability	Widely available
Conditions Tested For	Down's Syndrome
	Edward's Syndrome
	spina bifida
	anencephaly
Risks Posed by the Test	None
Options: if high risk	amniocentesis
	high resolution ultrasound scan
	do nothing

4

Ultrasound Scans

Most women expect to have one or two ultrasound scans during their pregnancy. Research tells us that parents like scans and feel more attached to their babies as a result of them.

> 'It's helped the baby to have an identity for me – and certainly for my husband.'

> *Balbinder*

Fathers, in particular, seem to find that seeing their baby on the screen makes the pregnancy more real for them. The psychological impact of scanning appears, therefore, to be very positive although there may be occasions when having seen your baby on an ultrasound scan makes a miscarriage or a decision to end your pregnancy even harder.

'It almost made it harder seeing that Lydia was OK, moving around and the heartbeat and everything, and then losing her five weeks later.'

Janine

Long-term Effects of Ultrasound Scans

There are still questions to be answered about the possible long-term side-effects of ultrasound scans. When scanning was first introduced in America, women were scanned as often as once a week simply to 'have a look at the baby'. At that time, it seemed very unlikely that babies could be harmed by ultrasound but, since then, some studies have suggested that scanning may affect babies in ways that we don't really understand. Research carried out in Scandinavia showed that babies whose mothers had a lot of scans during their pregnancies were more likely to be left-handed than babies whose mothers had no scans or only one. Whilst there's nothing at all wrong with being left-handed, the fact that so many more children than is usual turned out to be left-handed made doctors wonder whether their brains had been affected in some way by the scans their mothers had had. However, another study found no difference between the performance at school of children who had been scanned before birth and those who hadn't.

Saying 'No' to a Scan

Today, scans are treated a little more cautiously than they were years ago in America and while it's still routine for women to have one or two, they are no longer done just because it's fun to have a look at the baby. However, the vast majority of hospitals do expect that every woman will have one scan during her pregnancy and if you decide that you don't want to be scanned, you may find that your doctor and midwife are very surprised.

'I decided not to have a scan – every time I visited the hospital Antenatal Clinic, they expected to routinely scan me and some staff got very cross with me when I refused. In the end, I avoided the hospital and only attended my local GP clinic.'

Wendy

'Having read up on the subject of ultrasound scans, I was not convinced that the scans had been proved safe to my satisfaction. I felt it was a risk I was unwilling to take and decided not to have a scan. This led to a tremendous amount of pressure from the health professionals which I felt led to a huge amount of stress during my pregnancy.'

Louise

If you are certain that you don't want a scan, say so clearly to your midwife and ask her to make a note in your maternity records so that other health professionals caring for you will know where you stand. It is your choice whether or not to have a scan and no one should *assume* that you will have one.

How Effective Is Ultrasound Scanning?

It's important to understand that there are a large number of factors which influence how much your scan can tell you about your baby. Scans certainly don't pick up every problem, even very major ones, which babies might have. Small problems are frequently missed and sometimes abnormalities are picked up which appear to have corrected themselves by the time your baby is born. For instance, you may be told that your baby's kidneys don't seem quite normal or that your baby's heart has a slightly odd appearance, yet your baby has no problems with either his heart or his kidneys after birth.

Weeks of Pregnancy	What the Scan Might Show
up to 13 weeks	– how many weeks pregnant you are
	– how many babies you are carrying
	– whether your baby's heart is beating
	– anencephaly
	– very major problems with the way the baby's body and limbs have developed
18–22 weeks	– spina bifida and hydrocephalus
	– anencephaly
	– major heart and kidney problems
	– problems with your baby's stomach and digestive tract
30 weeks and later	– minor problems such as cleft lip
	– some heart problems missed at the 20 weeks scan
	– minor kidney problems

Sometimes women are told when they have an early scan that their baby has a cystic hygroma. This is a watery tumour on the neck.

A cystic hygroma may be associated with conditions such as Down's Syndrome or it may mean nothing at all. Your doctor will invite you to have another scan later on to check the cyst by which time it might well have disappeared. Being told that your baby has a swelling on his or her neck is bound to cause you a lot of anxiety. It's your decision whether to have another scan during your pregnancy or to take no further action.

> 'The doctor told us there was a "bright spot" in the baby's bowels and two cysts at the back of the baby's neck and that research has shown that these two symptoms combined often point to the strong possibility of Down's Syndrome. She strongly recommended an amniocentesis and said we should start thinking about a termination.
>
> 'We decided not to have any more tests. We saw the same doctor again when our (perfectly healthy) baby was scanned again six weeks after she was born to check up on the cysts. She didn't remember us at all. The cysts were gone "which is always the case" as she now said rather carelessly. I wish I had told her about the way we felt, but politeness and relief made us just smile politely.'
>
> *Zoe*

Even some very major problems will be missed. The following graph shows how successful ultrasound is in detecting major problems in unborn babies:

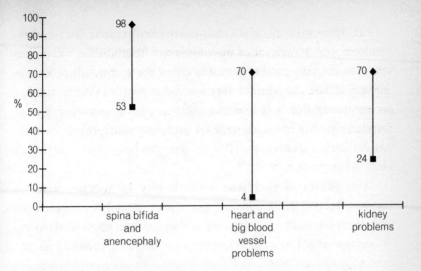

ULTRASOUND DETECTION RATES

The reason why such a wide-range of percentages is given is because the effectiveness of scans depends on such things as:

– the quality of the scanner
– the training the sonographer has received
– how good at scanning the sonographer is
– whether the mother is overweight
– what position the baby is lying in
– how long the scan lasts

Probably the most important of these factors is how long the scan lasts. A five minutes scan will only detect a few abnormalities whereas a 30 minutes scan has a much better chance of finding any problems which the baby might have. The second most important factor is the skill of the sonographer; some people have a 'knack' for scanning and some are simply much better trained than others.

Problems with the heart and major blood vessels are the most common abnormalities in newborn babies. Unfortunately, ultrasound scans are not very good at detecting these. Some hospitals pick up as few as 5 in 100 and even the very best hospitals with the most expert sonographers detect only about 70 in every 100. In other words, most of the time, most of the heart problems which babies have are not detected. Parents may feel that their scan has given them the 'all clear' when, in fact, it hasn't.

The quality of your scan depends to a very large extent on the hospital you go to. Some hospitals have much better equipment and invest far more in the training of their sonographers than others. A hospital attached to a university may detect as many as 77 per cent of major problems in babies whereas an average city hospital will find as few as 36 per cent. With enough money, it would probably be possible to achieve a 70 per cent detection rate throughout the country, but, given the financial situation of the National Health Service, it's not likely that scanning will become this good in the near future! So even if you go to the best maternity unit in the country with the highest rate of picking up problems on ultrasound, you still can't be certain that your doctors will find out everything about your baby.

What Does a Scan Involve?

If you have a scan very early in pregnancy, before thirteen weeks, you will be asked to drink as much as you can immediately beforehand so that your bladder is full. This is so that the bladder will push the uterus out of the pelvis. If the uterus remains inside the pelvis which is its normal position in the first weeks of pregnancy, the pelvic bones prevent it from being seen on the scan.

You will be asked to put on a hospital gown and to lie down. The sonographer will put some clear gel on your tummy which is cold and sticky and stains if it gets on your clothes – hence the gown! The gel improves the contact between your skin and the ultrasound-transducer. You may find that your full bladder makes you feel quite uncomfortable when the sonographer presses down on your tummy with the transducer. Try and distract yourself by looking at the pictures of your baby on the screen and asking as many questions as you want.

The sonographer should explain to you what she is looking for and help you to understand what you are seeing on the screen. You may be able to see your baby sucking, swallowing and making breathing movements. You may be able to see his stomach filling and the bladder emptying. You may be able to see him doing somersaults or even rolling his eyes depending on how far on in your pregnancy you are. You can ask to have a picture of your baby; (some hospitals charge a small fee for this).

Who Will the Sonographer Be?

Generally, the person who does your scan will be a radiographer whose training includes ultrasound scanning. He or she may or may not know a great deal about obstetrics. Sometimes the sonographer is a doctor and sometimes, although not very commonly, a midwife who has had special training in scanning. If your sonographer is a doctor or midwife, they may be able to tell you immediately the significance of what they are seeing on the scan. A radiographer, however, may need to ask someone else to interpret the scan if there appears to be an abnormality.

Abnormal Scans

Most women 'know' when the sonographer has found something wrong with their baby. The screen may be turned away from you so that you can't see the pictures any more or the person doing the scan may ask for a second opinion:

> 'I lay with the monitor facing me and it was suddenly turned away. The lady called for another radiographer who in turn looked and saw and called for the doctor who told me there was "nothing with a heartbeat".'

Emma

Some women simply sense a quietness in the room and feel that all is not well. If the person doing the scan is a radiographer rather than a doctor, he or she will probably not be allowed to give you bad news, but will have to refer you to your consultant. Even if your sonographer is a doctor or midwife, hospital policy may still dictate that the consultant be called. So just when your need for information is most urgent because you are aware that a problem has been found, you may find yourself kept in the dark until the consultant arrives.

If there seems to be a problem with your baby and you are having a scan at your GP's surgery or a small hospital where the equipment is not very sophisticated, you will probably be asked to go to a larger hospital for a more detailed scan. Insist that the appointment is as soon as possible because having to wait is very difficult.

'The abnormalities in our baby were first spotted when I went for my 20-week scan, although the doctor could not tell us what was wrong. I was confused and upset because the first scan at 16 weeks and all my blood tests were fine. I convinced myself that there had been some mistake because I felt so healthy and our baby was already a person to us ... The doctor said that he would make an appointment for a detailed scan at the maternity hospital 45 minutes away, and that I would get the appointment by post. I became very upset that I would have to wait and so he went to the phone and made the appointment there and then. In the event, I had to wait for a week because the diagnostic unit at the hospital was so busy. When I went for the detailed scan, Matt came with me. The doctors couldn't tell us for certain what was wrong. They said that the baby's head was a little on the large side and that there seemed to be a defect with his heart, but again they could not see enough to tell. The next five weeks were hell. We went back to the diagnostic unit a further four times. The staff there were wonderful – nothing was too much trouble, but it was so frustrating that they could not tell us what the abnormalities were. On our fifth visit, they arranged for us to see a paediatric cardiologist who looked and listened to our baby's heart through the ultrasound scan. He told us that our baby's heart was badly deformed.'

Liz
(SATFA News, *September 1996)*

When you have had a straightforward pregnancy and felt your baby kicking inside you, it comes as a tremendous shock to be told that there may be something wrong. Don't hesitate to ask for things to be repeated if you don't immediately understand. Make sure that you get all the information you need and then ask for time to consider your options.

Questions to Ask If Your Scan Shows a Problem

1 What exactly is the problem?
2 How serious is the problem?
3 What will it mean for my baby if he is born with this problem?
4 Are you quite sure about what the scan is showing?
5 Is there a better scanner in this or another hospital which could give a more detailed picture?
6 What are my options now?
7 How quickly do I have to make up my mind about what to do?

Scans at the End of Pregnancy

If you become anxious during the second half of your pregnancy that your baby is not moving around as much as she was, you can ask to have a scan to check that she is all right. In the last twelve weeks of pregnancy, a scan can measure how much amniotic fluid there is around your baby and how healthy the placenta is. If the amount of fluid is much more or less than normal, your baby could have a problem with swallowing or with her kidneys. If a serious problem is found or if the placenta appears to be failing and you are well on in your pregnancy, you will be offered either a caesarean section or an induction of labour so that your baby can be born and receive the treatment she needs.

Scanning the Placenta

Scans are also used to look at the placenta and to check that it's not so low in the womb that it will prevent your baby from being born. Although 20–30 per cent of women are told in the middle of pregnancy that their placenta is 'low-lying' and close to the neck of the womb where the baby has to come out, only about 0.5 per cent of these women still have a problem at the end of pregnancy. It's not that the placenta has moved; it's just that the lower part of the womb stretches as you become more heavily pregnant so that the placenta appears to be further away from the neck of the womb than it was before.

Measuring Blood Flow

In hospitals with very specialized scanners, it's possible to measure the blood flow in the umbilical arteries and through the placenta. If the results are abnormal, your doctor will want to monitor your baby's growth by scanning you regularly during the rest of your pregnancy.

Advantages of Ultrasound

❏ you can enjoy seeing your baby
❏ helps fathers feel closer to their babies
❏ a simple technique
❏ gives you reassurance
❏ provides immediate information about your baby

Disadvantages of Ultrasound

❏ may have long-term side-effects, as yet unknown
❏ how good your scan is depends on many factors outside your control
❏ may give you false reassurance

5

The Nuchal Translucency Test

As ultrasound scanning becomes more and more sophisticated, it seems likely that it will increasingly replace other forms of pregnancy screening. One of the newest antenatal tests, the nuchal translucency test, combines a specialized ultrasound scan with a blood test to estimate the risk of your baby having Down's Syndrome.

You can have the nuchal translucency test early on in pregnancy (at about the same time as you would have a CVS) to find out how likely it is that your baby will have Down's Syndrome. The test was developed at King's College Hospital by Professor Nicolaides who is well known for his work on pregnancy screening. The test is being carried out in about twenty hospitals in the south-east of England and you can have it privately at the Fetal Medicine Centre in London. It costs about £80 (plus however much it will cost you to travel to London).

Judith describes how she made the decision to have a nuchal translucency test:

'Being pregnant with my fourth child aged 39, I had to make my choice about prenatal testing. I felt I wanted to do *something*.

I have no known family history of Down's Syndrome or other serious genetic disorders, and three healthy children. Nevertheless, I felt that the blood test detection rate for Down's was not good enough for me (and particularly for my partner) ... Initially, therefore, I thought I would opt for amniocentesis. This was a reluctant decision, as I wasn't keen on the invasive aspect, either for myself or the baby ... The nuchal translucency test seemed an ideal option for me.'

(*Modern Midwife*, March 1997)

What Does the Test Involve?

The test simply involves having a detailed ultrasound scan using the most up-to-date equipment to get a 'high resolution' picture of your baby. The person who does the scan may be a sonographer (a specialist in ultrasound scanning) or a doctor trained in the nuchal translucency test. A thin layer of fluid between two folds of skin at the back of the baby's head is measured during the scan. Babies who have Down's Syndrome (and some less common genetic conditions) have a thicker layer of fluid behind their necks than unaffected babies.

'The surroundings were very relaxing and the doctor who carried out the scan was pleasant and helpful, answering all my questions fully. The measurement and observations took only about 10 minutes and I got a photograph of my baby.'

Glynnis

When estimating the risk of your baby having Down's Syndrome, her heart rate as well as the amount of fluid behind her neck is added into the calculations. Babies who have Down's Syndrome tend to have a much higher heart rate than babies who don't. The age of the mother is another important factor which is taken into account because a very young woman has a much lower risk of conceiving a baby with Down's Syndrome than an older woman. At the end of the test, you can be given an idea of your risk based on the ultrasound scan, your baby's heart rate and your age, but you will also be asked to have a blood test so that further information can be fed into the calculations. This means that you have to wait another four or five days to hear what the final estimation of your risk is.

Just occasionally, a woman is told immediately after the nuchal translucency test that she is at low risk of having a baby with Down's Syndrome only to be given a much higher risk later on after her blood results have also been taken into account. This is a very difficult situation for anyone to handle. You may have heaved a huge sigh of relief when your risk was first given to you, only to find that four days later, you have to think about whether to have more tests to try to find out if the lower or the higher risk is the more accurate.

Reliability of Nuchal Translucency Test

Although this test is relatively new, it does seem that it is very good at predicting which women are at the highest risk of being pregnant with Down's Syndrome babies. The test is more accurate for women over 35 years, but less so for younger women. This is because your age is taken into account as well as the test results when your risk of having a Down's Syndrome baby is calculated and the older you are, the higher your risk is.

Because the nuchal translucency test requires a really excellent ultrasound scanner, it's possible for the doctor to examine your baby minutely for any problems there might be with the development of his heart, stomach, bladder or kidneys at the same time as carrying out the nuchal measurement. Your doctor can also look at the development of your baby's brain and spine to check for anencephaly and spina bifida although, because the scan is carried out so early in your pregnancy, there's a limit to how much can be seen.

The Nuchal Translucency Test and Twins

This test is very helpful if you are pregnant with twins and want to find out whether your babies have Down's Syndrome. The two babies can be measured separately and you are given an estimate of the risk of Down's for each baby. You have to bear in mind that the test isn't quite as reliable for twins as it is for one baby because it's harder to interpret the blood test results which are also part of the nuchal translucency test when there are two babies to take into account.

The Future of the Nuchal Translucency Test

It's by no means certain that the nuchal translucency test will eventually be available to all women on the NHS. The test is time-consuming and requires very sophisticated equipment. This means that it's expensive and staff need to be highly trained in order to carry it out.

The problem with the nuchal translucency test is that, although it's pretty accurate, it doesn't tell you for certain whether your baby has Down's Syndrome. It's not a diagnostic test. This means that if you get a high risk result, you'll have to decide whether to go on to have another test such as chorionic villus sampling or amniocentesis if you want to find out for certain whether your baby has Down's. These tests carry a 0.5–2 per cent risk of miscarriage. If you have a positive result, you'll have to make a decision about whether to end your pregnancy. When you are thinking about early pregnancy testing, it's important to remember that nature itself tends to bring abnormal pregnancies to an end quite quickly and at least half the women pregnant with Down's Syndrome babies are destined to miscarry before 14 weeks.

This is perhaps the main problem with early pregnancy tests – they enable women to find out that their baby has a serious health problem at a time when nature itself may be working to bring the pregnancy to an end. Some people argue that if there was no early testing and nature was simply allowed to take its course, a lot of women would be spared the anxiety of trying to decide what to do when they find out their baby might have or does have Down's Syndrome. Other people argue that a test such as the nuchal translucency test puts women in the driving seat – they can make their own choices rather than simply waiting to see what happens.

Only you can decide how you feel.

Nuchal Translucency Test

Screening/Diagnostic	**Screening**
When Carried Out	10–14 weeks of pregnancy
Availability	Not widely available. Hospitals offering the the test are situated mainly in the southeast of England. The Fetal Medicine Centre in London offers the test privately (cost about £80)

Conditions Tested For	Down's Syndrome
	(Also: Edward's Syndrome
	Patau's Syndrome
	Turner's Syndrome
	anencephaly
	severe spina bifida)
Risks posed by the test itself	? (possible long-term side-effects of ultrasound scanning, as yet unknown)
Options – if the results suggest a high risk	chorionic villus sampling amniocentesis do nothing

Advantages of Nuchal Translucency Test

❑ an *early* pregnancy test
❑ you can see your baby on a high resolution scanner
❑ results available immediately

Disadvantages of Nuchal Translucency Test

❑ not generally available
❑ you may have to pay for it
❑ you could get two conflicting results
❑ early pregnancy testing may be inappropriate because many babies with genetic conditions and other problems miscarry anyway

6

Diagnostic Tests

Chorionic Villus Sampling (CVS)

Chorionic villus sampling (CVS) is the only diagnostic test which is widely available to women very early in their pregnancies. There is a risk that the baby will miscarry after the procedure. It's hard to quantify this risk as quite a few pregnancies end in miscarriage before they have reached fourteen weeks anyway. So a baby who miscarries following a CVS test may, in fact, have miscarried even if her mother had not had the test. Doctors think, however, that the miscarriage rate due to the test itself is between 0.5 and 2 per cent. This is an important factor for you to take into account when deciding whether or not you would like to have chorionic villus sampling. Some women feel that the risk of miscarriage is not acceptable to them:

'I'd had a bleed at eight weeks – a threatened miscarriage – and I'd heard that if you have a CVS test, there is a very small possibility that you might have a miscarriage from that and because I'd already had problems, I didn't want to risk anything.'

Lauren

You might feel, however, that the advantages of being able to have a diagnostic test very early on in pregnancy outweigh the small risk of miscarriage.

Miscarriage Following CVS

The miscarriage rate following CVS varies from hospital to hospital, from as few as 0.5 miscarriages per 100 tests at some hospitals to as many as 5 per 100 at others.

Ask your hospital to tell you what its miscarriage rate is. Many people feel that this information should be available to the public. If you're told that you are not entitled to know, you might ask yourself why the hospital is being so secretive.

The number of CVS tests a hospital carries out a year will have a big influence on its miscarriage rate. The more the hospital does, the better its results are likely to be.

In general, hospitals have to be doing more than a hundred CVS tests a year to be able to achieve a 0.5 miscarriage rate.

(All these points apply to amniocentesis as well.)

'I was very keen to have CVS because of being over 35 and because you can have it earlier in pregnancy than an amnio-centesis. If there was any problem and I did decide to go for a termination, I wanted that to be as early as possible. I had the test at 12 weeks.'

Polly

What Does the Test Involve?

If you choose to have a CVS test, you will probably be referred to a Regional Unit where the doctors are specialists in pregnancy testing.

The procedure starts with an ultrasound scan so that the doctor can see where the placenta is in your womb. He or she will then put a very fine needle through your tummy and take a tiny sample of the placenta. More rarely, the procedure may be carried out through the vagina and cervix. Try to relax while the procedure is being carried out – most women say that it's not painful:

'It wasn't comfortable, but it wasn't as bad as I'd expected.'

Yukiko

The sample is sent away to a medical laboratory for examination and you should receive the results within 7 to 10 days. Remember that a CVS test cannot tell you whether your baby has spina bifida but only whether he has a genetic condition such as Down's Syndrome. You may therefore want to have some further testing later on in your pregnancy to check that your baby's limbs and insides have developed normally and this means thinking about a blood test (see Chapter 3) when you are about 16 weeks pregnant and/or an ultrasound scan (see Chapter 4) when you are about 20 weeks pregnant.

Chorionic Villus Sampling

Screening/Diagnostic	Diagnostic
Availability	Available at teaching hospitals and some smaller maternity units
When Carried Out	Around 11 weeks of pregnancy
Conditions Tested For	Down's Syndrome (also: Edward's Syndrome Patau's Syndrome Turner's Syndrome)
Risks Posed by the Test Itself	0.5–2% risk of miscarriage
Options: positive diagnosis	Have a scan later in pregnancy to check the baby for any other problems End the pregnancy

CVS may give inconclusive results and you may have to have a retest.

Amniocentesis

During pregnancy, your baby is protected by a bubble of fluid in which he floats. This fluid is called amniotic fluid, or liquor, or sometimes simply 'the waters'. The waters contain cells shed from your baby and these cells can be tested by a medical laboratory to see whether the baby has Down's Syndrome. The laboratory can also diagnose other conditions which your baby might have.

Generally, you have an amniocentesis when you are about 18 weeks pregnant. You may have to wait three to four weeks for the results which means that by the time you get them, you will be able to feel your baby moving quite noticeably inside you. This makes the decision about whether to have a termination if the baby does have Down's Syndrome extremely traumatic.

Before deciding whether to have an amniocentesis, it's important to understand that only about 50 per cent of the genetic abnormalities which the test detects are due to Down's Syndrome. Your amniocentesis may show that your baby does not have Down's Syndrome but does have some much rarer genetic problem. Occasionally, babies are found to have genetic conditions which doctors know very little about, and your consultant may not be able to tell you how seriously such a condition will affect your baby or whether it will affect him at all. Many people think that amniocentesis is only for Down's Syndrome, and don't realize that when the laboratory examines the fluid taken from the mother, it may come up with all sorts of unexpected results.

Questions to Ask

Ask your hospital how long it will be before you get the results of your amniocentesis. Nowadays, a really good lab will be able to get the results back to the hospital in 9 to 10 days.

Also ask your hospital what its miscarriage rate is following amniocentesis. This is something you need to take into account when you are thinking about this test. There is a risk that the procedure will disturb the pregnancy and that you will miscarry your baby afterwards. Hospitals which carry out lots of amnios will probably have a miscarriage rate as low as 0.5 per 100 procedures. Hospitals which don't do many amnios may well have a higher rate, perhaps up to 2 miscarriages per 100 procedures or even more.

What's Involved

Before you have an amniocentesis, you are asked to make sure that your bladder is empty. You will then be continuously scanned while your doctor puts a long needle through the wall of your tummy into your womb and withdraws about 20 ml of fluid. The scan picture helps the doctor to avoid the placenta and to find a pool of fluid for the sample. For most women, having an amniocentesis isn't uncomfortable:

'The amnio was OK; it wasn't painful or anything – I just felt a push as the needle went in.'

Sara

Some women find the procedure more traumatic perhaps because they are so anxious.

'Damian was with me throughout the test. The feeling of contraction as the needle goes in and comes out was very strange although I had been told to expect it. I was told to rest for 24 hours afterwards – I felt totally emotionally drained.'

Petra

After the amniocentesis, the doctor will listen to your baby's heart to make sure that he is all right. If your blood group is Rhesus negative, you will be given an injection of 'anti-D' so that you don't react to any of your baby's red blood cells which might have got into your circulation during the amniocentesis (see Chapter 2). Before you go home, you will have the chance to rest for an hour at the hospital and your midwife will advise you to spend the next 48 hours quietly at home. This is to minimize the risk of a miscarriage which is most likely to happen within a couple of days of the amniocentesis.

It can seem a very long couple of days while you wait to see whether your baby will be OK. After this, you have another long wait of up to three weeks before you get the results of the test. For most women, this is a very difficult period and it is almost impossible to concentrate on anything. Some women find that the only way they can cope is to have a programme for each day which means that they never have a free moment to think about themselves. Some are panicked every time the phone or the doorbell rings because they are so frightened of receiving bad news.

> 'If the result had been positive, then my GP would've arrived unannounced on the doorstep, so for at least the last week of the three weeks' wait, I was a gibbering idiot every time someone knocked on the door.'

> *Dorcas*

Amniocentesis for Twins

Apart from the nuchal translucency test which isn't generally available on the NHS, amniocentesis is the only other test that's helpful for diagnosing Down's Syndrome when the mother is pregnant with two babies. If each baby is floating in his own bubble of amniotic fluid, it's possible for the doctor to take a sample of the fluid from each bubble.

The two samples are then sent to the laboratory for testing and the results can tell you whether one or both or neither of your babies has Down's. However, before you decide to go ahead with an amniocentesis, it's really important to think what you will do if just one baby is found to have Down's. It is possible to have what's called a 'selective termination' when just one baby is aborted, but it's fair to say that most women (and staff) find this a very traumatic procedure.

Double amniocentesis is generally only offered at Regional Referral Centres where the doctors have a lot of experience in carrying out the procedure. Very occasionally, both the babies in a twin pregnancy are lying in the same bubble of water. If this is the case, there's no point in having an amniocentesis because the test won't be able to distinguish between the two babies.

Early Amniocentesis

You might think that it would be better if you could have an amniocentesis much earlier in pregnancy, say before 14 weeks and before you have felt your baby moving. Early amniocentesis has been tried, but it doesn't seem to have many advantages over chorionic villus sampling. When amniocentesis is carried out very early in pregnancy, the results for spina bifida are not at all reliable so it's not better than CVS in this respect. Mid-pregnancy amniocentesis can diagnose spina bifida as well as Down's Syndrome. At a Regional Referral Unit where the doctors are very skilled at carrying out CVS and amniocentesis, there is little difference in the miscarriage rates following the two procedures and CVS is preferable to amniocentesis because you'll probably get the results sooner.

The advantage of early amniocentesis over chorionic villus sampling is that it may be a slightly more reliable test. Just occasionally, a mistake is made during the CVS test so that it's not the baby's tissue which is sampled, but the mother's. The results are then wrongly interpreted as applying to the baby when really they're giving information about the mother's genetic make-up. Amniocentesis doesn't run the risk of this particular error. However, early amniocentesis is a tricky procedure; it can be difficult for the doctor to collect enough fluid from around the baby and the fluid which is collected may not contain any of the baby's cells. After waiting a few weeks for the result, you could find that you're being told the test wasn't successful and that you need to think about having another amniocentesis or choosing a screening test such as the triple test.

Amniocentesis

Screening/Diagnostic	Diagnostic
When Carried Out	13–18 weeks of pregnancy
Availability	*Early* amniocentesis not widely available; otherwise, amniocentesis generally available
Conditions Tested For	Down's Syndrome (also Patau's Syndrome Edward's Syndrome Turner's Syndrome Other Syndromes spina bifida anencephaly)
Risks Posed by the Test	Small possibility of miscarriage afterwards (0.5%–2%)
Your Options: positive diagnosis	do nothing end the pregnancy

Cordocentesis

If you have a scan in the second half of pregnancy and your doctor can see that your baby has certain problems which are often linked to conditions such as Down's or Edward's Syndrome, she may suggest to you that you have a cordocentesis to get a firm diagnosis. The advantage of cordocentesis over amniocentesis is that the results are available within 72 hours instead of your having to wait a couple of weeks. You will probably have to go to a Regional Referral Centre to have the test because it's quite a tricky procedure. A doctor takes some blood from your baby's umbilical cord, using ultrasound to guide the needle. The procedure carries about a 1.5 per cent risk of miscarriage afterwards.

Advantages of Amniocentesis

- ❏ It's diagnostic and can tell you for certain whether your baby has Down's Syndrome (or other rarer genetic conditions).

Disadvantages of Amniocentesis

- ❏ 0.5–2% risk of miscarriage
- ❏ May damage the placenta, leading to bleeding
- ❏ May cause infection in the mother
- ❏ May detect a condition other than Down's Syndrome which doctors don't know much about

7

Terminating Your Pregnancy

If the results of a diagnostic test show that your baby has a serious disabling condition, you will be offered an abortion. Even if you are convinced that this is the right course to take and that it is best for your baby, your own physical and mental health and your relationship with your partner, you may still feel guilty:

> 'With the full extent of abnormalities confirmed, we really felt that we had no choice but to opt for a termination. Needless to say, our emotions were in turmoil; shock, heartbreak, disappointment, and the underlying sense of guilt at having taken this awful decision to deprive our baby of life.'

> *Janine*
> (SATFA News, *March 1997*)

You need to understand exactly how the termination will be carried out and how long it will take you to recover afterwards. Your hospital should have a specially trained nurse or midwife who can answer your questions and give you the support you deserve. Being well prepared will help you cope better with what is going to happen.

Termination of Pregnancy Before 14 Weeks

If you are less than 14 weeks pregnant, you will probably be admitted to a gynaecology ward where there will be women waiting for a variety of operations which may have nothing to do with pregnancy. Most of these women will not be going through the same kind of emotional upheaval as you are and it can be very difficult to be on a ward where there are other people laughing and joking and watching television when you are going through such a sad time. There may be other women who are booked to have a termination of pregnancy or there may just be you. Ask if your partner or a relative or friend can stay with you until you are taken down to theatre if that is what you want.

Very often, an early termination of pregnancy will be carried out as a day case which means that you will be admitted to hospital in the morning, have the operation and, provided that you are well, be discharged home in the evening. You will be asked not to eat anything on the day of the operation and just before going to theatre, you will need to take off your make-up and remove your jewellery. If you have a special ring, you will be able to keep it on your finger provided it is covered with tape. When you go down to theatre for the termination, you will have some electrodes attached to your chest to monitor your heart during the operation.

An anaesthetist will give you an injection into your arm to put you to sleep. The operation itself is quite a short one and simply involves stretching the neck of your womb and removing the contents. This is called a D&E which stands for 'Dilatation' (opening the neck of the womb) and 'Evacuation' (removing the contents of the womb). When you wake up again, a nurse will be with you to check your blood pressure and ensure that you are not bleeding heavily from the vagina.

You should be able to go home later the same day. Do think about who is going to take you home as you shouldn't drive immediately after an operation or have to walk for a bus. You also need to arrange for someone to look after you for a couple of days. Having a general anaesthetic will probably make you feel 'not quite with it' for a while and you will be grieving for the loss of your baby:

'I was booked in for the termination 48 hours later ... It was all over so quickly ... The next day, Friday, I experienced a great sense of relief as the bleeding was very slight, the nausea disappeared, my appetite returned, and my GP paid a very welcome home visit. I probably seemed too euphoric as I praised the care I had received. He kindly warned me of the grief and sadness which would follow. I insisted I was fit enough to return to work the following Monday ... A great wave of sadness came the very same night, as I realized I had no place to put my grief. I didn't know whether the baby had been a boy or a girl. I couldn't put a name to my sadness. I didn't know who I was grieving for ... There is that need to cry and cry, and it does bring some relief and clarity.'

Jayne
(SATFA News, *March 1996*)

Termination of Pregnancy Using Mifepristone (RU486)

If you are very early on in your pregnancy, you may be able to avoid having a general anaesthetic for a termination. Some obstetricians are using a drug called Mifepristone which is taken by mouth. You will be given the tablets at the hospital and asked to return two days later in order to have some prostaglandin pessaries which a nurse or midwife will place high up in your vagina. The pessaries melt and soften the cervix or neck of the womb which makes the womb contract so that your body itself ends the pregnancy.

Termination Later in Pregnancy

If you are more than 14 weeks pregnant when you make the decision to end your pregnancy, you will have either a medical or a surgical termination, depending on your hospital's protocol. You may be attending a hospital where you will be given the choice and it's important to understand what each method involves.

Medical Termination

Medical termination is the most usual way of ending a pregnancy after 14 weeks. Drugs are used to help your body go into labour and then to expel the contents of your womb. This is a much more traumatic procedure than having an early termination and you need to:

- think about who would be the best person to go into hospital to support you through the labour
- find out exactly what will happen while you are in hospital

    – think about whether you want to see or hold your baby after he
      or she is delivered

Some hospitals induce labour on the gynaecology ward and some on
the labour ward. You will have a pessary placed in your vagina every
three hours up to fifteen hours or until the termination is complete.
The pessaries contain prostaglandins which soften the neck of the
womb and stimulate your body to go into labour. Sometimes, prostaglandins are given by a drip into your arm.

After your baby has been delivered, you will be given an injection
of a drug called syntometrine which helps your womb contract strongly to push out the placenta (afterbirth) and ensure that you don't
bleed heavily. If by any chance, some of the placenta is left behind in
your womb, you will need to have a local or general anaesthetic so that
the womb can be emptied surgically.

Because it's not natural for your body to go into labour so early
in pregnancy, it can be difficult to induce labour. Labour can be very
painful and may last quite a long time. There is no need for you
to suffer a lot of pain. Your midwife will offer you pain-killers such
as paracetamol or codeine tablets to take by mouth or injections of
stronger drugs such as diamorphine or pethidine to help you cope
with the pain. These drugs can be given every four hours.

Some women punish themselves for ending their pregnancy by
refusing any pain relief. Their sense of guilt is not necessarily shared
by other women also having a termination or not expressed in the
same way. You cannot change your feelings and shouldn't be afraid
that your reactions are unhealthy:

'I was given a pessary at about midday and another at about 3 p.m. I was on Ward 7 in a private en suite room, and I felt strangely relaxed until things started to happen. The worst pain was when my waters broke. I had no pain relief although it was offered – I felt I wasn't entitled to it.'

Katie
(SATFA News, March 1977)

When your baby is born, you may feel that under no circumstances do you want to see him or her or even to be told the sex. You might feel that you simply want the baby to be taken away as quickly as possible and to close your mind to what has happened. You might be frightened to see your baby in case he or she looks very deformed. All these feelings are understandable, but the vast majority of parents find that seeing and holding their baby is an immense comfort. If you see your baby, you know that you are grieving for a real little person whom you love and have had great expectations for. You have an individual to attach your grief to and this seems to help people recover better than if they try to deny their baby ever existed.

It is extremely unlikely that your baby's appearance will upset you. Generally, the baby looks very normal and peaceful although the skin may be quite red. When she is born, your midwife will clean her gently and wrap her in a blanket before bringing her to you and your partner to see and, if you wish, hold:

'They gave her to us and I was almost afraid to look – I had imagined a grotesque, deformed body but she looked so beautiful.'

Samantha
(SATFA News, September 1996)

Advantages of Medical Termination

❑ You don't have to have a general anaesthetic.
❑ You experience labour – some women feel that this is very important for them.
❑ You can see and hold your baby afterwards.
❑ A post-mortem can be carried out to find out exactly what the problem with the baby was.

Disadvantages

❑ The termination may take a long time – perhaps up to 18 hours.
❑ The drugs used sometimes cause sickness and diarrhoea.
❑ The labour may be painful.

If you choose not to see your baby, your midwife will probably take a picture and you may decide at a later date that you would like to have the photo. If you ring the hospital, the photo can be taken from your records and given to you. Some hospitals make a print of your baby's foot for you to keep. For many parents, little remembrances of their baby are extremely important to help them acknowledge what they have lost. Friends and relatives may avoid talking about the baby because they don't know what to say and you need to have some sort of confirmation that you were pregnant, that you did have a baby and that your baby died.

'Our dear Simon was wrapped in a blanket and a little hat by the midwife, Tracey, and I am very grateful now that we at least held him and Tracey took some pictures which I have in a treasured album.'

Louise
(SATFA News, *March 1977*)

Surgical Termination

Some hospitals use the same procedure for terminations carried out between 13 and 22 weeks as for an early termination. You have a general anaesthetic and the surgeon opens the neck of the womb and removes the baby with forceps. An ultrasound scan is used to guide the surgeon while performing the operation to ensure that the instruments being used for the termination don't damage your womb.

If you have a surgical termination, you will not be able to see your baby after you wake up. However, your hospital may have other ways of helping you grieve. For example, you may be able to write the name of your baby in a special Remembrance Book. Even if you don't want to do this immediately, you can go to the hospital weeks or even months later if you subsequently decide you want to record your baby's name and date of birth. Some hospitals hold a special service once a month for parents who have lost their babies and this gives people a chance to see that their grief is shared by others.

Advantages of Surgical Termination

❏ You will be asleep for the termination.
❏ The procedure is quick and you will probably not have to stay in hospital overnight.

Disadvantages

❏ You will not be able to see or hold your baby after the termination.
❏ There will probably be no post-mortem.
❏ There is some risk of damage to the cervix and uterus which might cause problems in another pregnancy.

Twin Pregnancies Where One Baby Has an Abnormality

If you are pregnant with twins and one of your babies is found to have a serious abnormality, it is possible to carry out what is called a 'selective termination'. This involves giving the affected baby a lethal injection into the heart. It is a risky procedure because sometimes the healthy baby is damaged too and both babies may miscarry afterwards. If you choose to have this kind of termination, you will naturally be very anxious about the well-being of your healthy baby:

'The consultant was extremely kind and courteous and talked to us and gave us lots of time. There was a small risk of miscarriage but we knew without question that we wanted to go ahead. We had to put our faith in him and his high reputation. But I couldn't help thinking that night, "What if they get the wrong baby?" We went back the following day for the termination. The baby's heart was injected and it was instantaneous and afterwards, they immediately showed me the other baby moving about and obviously unaffected. I was very upset. I had to sweat it out for three more days until they phoned me with the results of a blood sample they had taken from the aborted baby to say that yes, the baby had got Down's. For the rest of my pregnancy, I needed constant reassurance about the other baby.'

Emily

Getting the Support You Need

If you decide to end your pregnancy because your baby has a serious abnormality, you will need lots of support. Although to begin with, you may feel that you simply want to hide away and not talk to anybody, you will eventually feel a need to share your feelings with other people and to have the enormity of what you are going through acknowledged. Sadly, it may be hard for you to find people who are good at listening. Many of us are embarrassed by grief. We don't know what to say to people who have suffered a bereavement and we are frightened of saying the wrong thing so we avoid the sensitive issues which we fear may provoke emotions we can't handle. You will meet many people who simply won't be able to discuss the termination you have recently had. It's hard not to feel very let down by people who ignore your situation when all you want to do is talk about your pregnancy and your baby and your feelings. Try to identify two or three people who will listen and sympathize without trying to make you 'pull yourself together'. Try to remember that if your partner's not listening to you, it's probably because he's feeling as terrible as you are and is in as much need of support.

Grieving for the loss of a baby takes many different forms. To begin with, you and your partner may simply be unable to believe that you are not going to have a baby after all. You may feel very angry with God, the hospital, each other, everyone. You may feel that you will never be able to take up the threads of your everyday lives again because you no longer have the energy to do anything. You may feel that you want to see nobody at first, and then, later on, that you want to talk all the time about your loss. Quite often, couples find that their grief is 'out of sync'. One of the two is at the stage of wanting to withdraw from friends and family while the other is experiencing a strong need to talk and to share their grief openly. Both then feel that their partner isn't in sympathy with their needs and doesn't care about how they feel.

A man may find that the ending of a pregnancy which lasted only three or four months, before he could feel the baby kicking through his partner's tummy, has less impact on him than on his partner. This is not surprising. He has not been through the intense physical and emotional changes which his partner has been experiencing right from the very start of her pregnancy. Men sometimes find it difficult to understand how much an early miscarriage or abortion affects women and whilst some have been as deeply involved in the early weeks of the pregnancy as their partner, for others, it was never quite 'real'.

Men may also feel that they need to be strong for their partners and that they should hide their emotions. An American booklet for bereaved fathers advises:

'Don't try to be strong for your wife. Grieve with her. Grieving can be less difficult for those couples who can share in the emotions of the grief process. You may also be able to share your sadness with a close friend or acquaintance. You may be surprised to learn that many men have gone through similar experiences and are quite willing to talk with you if given the opportunity.'

(Grief and the Loss of Your Baby, *Rose Medical Center, Denver, Colorado, USA*)

Because there are so many different emotions involved in losing a baby and because the mother and father may experience even the same ones in different ways and at different stages, having a termination can sometimes cause a serious rift between couples:

'I carried on being supportive as at this stage my wife could not stand the sight of babies, pregnant women or anything associated with babies – and they're everywhere. It didn't affect me so it was up to me to do the shopping, hoovering, sort out the nursery. Slowly, arguments began to get worse. After a fortnight, we spoke to the SATFA (Support Around Termination For Abnormality) rep. When she arrived, I disappeared into the kitchen to make the tea and silently broke down. We were slowly getting further apart. I didn't know why and I had lost control.'

Jason
(SATFA News, *March 1996*)

It's important to try and keep talking to each other, or if this just isn't happening, to ask for help from someone else. There are several people and organizations you could contact:

- the Bereavement Counsellor at the hospital where you had the termination
- Relate (Relate used to be called the Marriage Guidance Council)
- SATFA (Support Around Termination For Abnormality)
- CRUSE, an organization that supports anyone in grief
- someone you know who has also had a termination
- a minister of your religion if you think he or she will be non-judgemental

In time, your hurt will become less although it's probably true to say that it will never entirely go away. Women who have had a miscarriage or a termination or who have given birth to a baby who died will talk about the experience twenty years later as if it happened yesterday. The majority, however, survive and move on in their lives:

'I can't face the fear of being pregnant for a while yet, but at least I can imagine a time to come when I might face it.'

Tracy
(SATFA News, September, 1996)

Lauren's story illustrates how the anguish of having a termination can change with the passing of time into acceptance and a new capacity to enjoy life and value it.

'Having suffered two miscarriages in the previous 12 months, I felt an optimistic 'third time lucky' when an early scan showed a healthy heartbeat but then after a routine scan at 20 weeks, I was taken into the consultant's office and given the devastating news that our baby was severely deformed –

no right leg at all, the right arm terminating at the elbow – only the left arm was normal. I was given the options available – termination or full support if I decided to continue.

'Later at home, my husband and I discussed the problem at length – I found myself praying to have a miscarriage when I had spent the previous 20 weeks praying not to. It was then that I realized what was the right decision for us. I just didn't want the responsibility of being the one to make it.

'We went into the hospital that afternoon and I was induced the following morning. I was left on the gynae ward for the majority of the labour which I later found out had been very upsetting for the other patients on the ward – many had been in tears for much of the day. I think it would have been better if I had been taken over to the labour ward earlier.

'The consultant had promised me that there would be no need to endure any pain as it would be better for the baby if I had any drugs available.

'This didn't prove to be the case – sometimes I felt that I couldn't bear the pain any longer – I was eventually put onto a morphine drip. It didn't seem to ease the pain. I just seemed to float in and out of consciousness as each contraction hit. Apparently, for the last couple of hours, they were just 30 seconds apart.

'Our daughter Annie was born just after 9 p.m. They gave her to us and I was almost afraid to look – I had imagined a grotesque deformed body but she looked so beautiful. I looked at her limbs, but she was so lovely. I can barely remember them – only the beautiful face – it was like looking in a mirror – she looked just like me! They took her away to photograph her and she came back in a small Moses basket dressed in a woollen hat and covered in a blanket. One of my biggest regrets is that she was photographed like this – only her face showing as though her deformities should be hidden. I would rather have had a photo of her as she was.

'Following the post-mortem, we held a small, private funeral at our local church. She was buried in the Garden of Remembrance. I don't visit the grave. Annie isn't there – she's in our hearts and with us forever.

'The next few months were very difficult. In addition to the pain of losing a child, I felt a failure as a woman – after all, having babies was something any woman could do, wasn't it? – anyone but me, it seemed!

'On the day that Annie was due, one of my best friends gave birth to a girl and it hurt so much. I was asked to be her godmother and as I held her, it seemed to help. It also had the effect of making me want to try again. A month later, I was pregnant for the fourth time and I tried to look forward to this baby – I was so scared!

'Our son was born a month prematurely and I loved him instantly.

'One morning, when he was about 3 months old, I woke up and realized that it was all over – I could parcel up the previous 20 months and call it a period of my life – but it was all over. I have a wonderful husband, a beautiful son and life was more than worth living again – I was happy!

'We'll never forget Annie – it still makes me sad some-times but the pain has gone. I don't think I ever thought that I'd get here but now that I have, I realize that the journey has made me a better person. I'm more compassionate, have more time to listen to other people's problems and I think I've got my priorities straighter. My desires are much simpler these days – my home and family are all that matter.'

Lauren
(SATFA News, September 1996)

Following a Termination of Pregnancy

Call your GP or the hospital if you have any of these problems. You might have an infection and this should be treated as soon as possible.

1 Vaginal bleeding which doesn't tail off after a few days
   or which suddenly gets heavier
   or which continues longer than a week
2 If you pass any large blood clots
3 If you feel feverish or unwell
4 If you have pains in your pelvis
5 If it stings to pass urine or your urine is foul smelling

8

Choosing to Keep Your Baby

The last chapter described the feelings of women who made the very difficult decision to end their pregnancies after finding out that their babies had serious abnormalities. Very often, it seems as if the whole thrust of antenatal testing is to ensure that babies who have health problems are prevented from being born. Sometimes, women find that they are refused diagnostic tests unless they agree *in advance* to have a termination should their baby prove to have Down's Syndrome or spina bifida or some other serious condition. Women may then feel they have to be deceitful in order to get the test they want:

'My obstetrician made it clear that it was worth me having an amniocentesis provided that we would go for a termination. And I said, "Fine," although I hadn't really decided. I reserved judgement to decide later and say, "Sorry, I'm going ahead with my pregnancy." '

Tina
(Being Pregnant, Giving Birth by Mary Nolan, page 54)

Some women feel very angry that there is an assumption that everyone will want to end their pregnancy if test results are unfavourable:

'I think it is the most shocking aspect of antenatal "care" that the government/medical profession puts such a priority on checking whether babies meet their standards of acceptability and, if not, promoting abortion. The information on screening tests makes it quite clear that this is the aim if a condition in the baby is discovered.'

Jacqui

'I find the emphasis on abortion as the main option should you find yourself carrying a child with Down's Syndrome, or even a hare lip, alarming and unethical.'

Rosemary

Others feel that the baby should be considered under no obligation to be 'perfect':

'I specifically asked not to be offered tests and the hospital was very understanding. This is a long awaited IVF baby. It is our responsibility to be good parents, not the baby's to be perfect.'

Tiara

Women who have already given birth to a disabled child may feel that they would not terminate a pregnancy if another baby was found to have the same disability because to do so would devalue the child they already have. They feel that ending the pregnancy would say to their existing child that his condition is unacceptable to them.

Some women are certain in their own minds that they would opt for a termination until they actually have to make that decision:

> 'I went in to the meeting with the consultant fairly sure that I was going to ask for a termination. During the meeting, the consultant didn't give me any advice. I thought he would tell me what to do. And by the end of the meeting, I wasn't so sure any more and I asked for another day to consider what I wanted to do.'

> *Natalie*

It's important to remember, whatever pressure you feel you are under from hospital staff or from friends and relatives, that you can decide to keep your baby even if she has been diagnosed as having a serious health problem. Just as there are excellent organizations to support women and couples who decide to opt for termination, so there are also organizations which will support you in your decision to continue your pregnancy. See the addresses section at the end of this book.

Two Women's Stories

Helen's and Nicole's stories illustrate the range of reasons why people decide to continue their pregnancies even when they know that they will give birth to disabled babies.

> 'I had the Double Test when I was 16 weeks into my third pregnancy. I thought it was a test for spina bifida; I didn't know it was a test for Down's Syndrome as well. So when someone from the hospital – I don't know who it was – rang

me a fortnight later and told me I had a 1 in 15 chance of having a baby with Down's, I didn't even connect what she wassaying to the test. I was booked for a scan on the Friday – I don't know what that was for either – and then told I should come into the hospital on Monday to have an amniocentesis.

'I was in a state of complete shock. Whatever it was that was happening shouldn't have been happening to me, it should have been happening to somebody else. The midwife whom I saw after the scan didn't seem to have much more idea about what was going on than I did or perhaps I just couldn't take in what she was saying.

'Over the weekend, I tried to think about what I would do if the baby definitely had Down's. I presumed that when I went into the hospital on the Monday, there would be some-body to counsel me and I took comfort from the thought that I would have the chance to talk things through before I had the amniocentesis. But when I got to the hospital, I was sim-ply told straightaway to get onto the table. It was obvious that the amnio was going to go ahead immediately. I tried to indi-cate that there were some questions I'd like to ask, but the doctor told me that if I wasn't going to terminate the preg-nancy if the baby had Down's, there was no point in having an amniocentesis.

'I was so confused that I simply let them get on with it. After the procedure, I was told to sit down for 20 minutes to rest and then that the results would come through in about three weeks time.

'It was during those weeks that I did some serious think-ing. I contacted the Down's Syndrome Association and talked to people there and they sent me booklets about Down's. I talked to my husband who said that the decision about whether to have the baby was mine and that he'd support me whichever way I went. Gradually, I came to the conclusion that I wanted to have this baby.

'After I got the amniocentesis result which was positive for Down's, I went to the hospital with my husband and we explained that we had decided to go ahead with the pregnancy. Our decision was accepted but I wasn't offered any support during the rest of my pregnancy. I was just treated like all the other women, although I felt quite different from them and was in a very different situation. My GP didn't help when I saw him. He told me that it would be best to end the pregnancy and said I should think what was best for my other two children.

'When I started in labour, I wondered just briefly whether I'd done the right thing in going ahead with the pregnancy, but as soon as Catherine was born, I knew I had. And I've never once wished I'd had an abortion since then. Catherine's four now.

'The support I received was much better after Catherine's birth. The paediatrician whom we saw was really excellent – very kind and understanding. Catherine had some serious heart problems – not uncommon in Down's Syndrome babies – and had to have surgery, but she's fine now. The paediatrician helped us through this and I also had support from my community midwife whose own sister has Down's. The Down's Syndrome Association put me in touch with the mother of a little boy with Down's and she helped me through the first weeks and months of Catherine's life and was a real friend.

'Catherine's simply a part of our family. My two boys are very protective towards her. She's just started school and she's an ordinary little school girl. She has friends and goes out to play with the other children, and she's learning to count and read. I expect her to learn how to look after herself and hopefully, she has the potential to get a job when she's grown up. I think I'm so lucky to have her and I don't think Down's Syndrome is so awful. You can't do an antenatal test for autism but that's much more upsetting than Down's and I do think I would have found it hard to cope with an autistic child.

'If I was advising someone who'd got a high risk test result, I'd say – make sure you get the full story. Talk to people; talk to the Down's Syndrome Association; get some books. The picture painted by the doctors is too negative. They're hell bent on getting women to terminate pregnancies when the tests are positive for Down's. I'd say to the woman that having a Down's child is OK and that she could consider having the baby adopted rather than ending the pregnancy. No one ever suggests to you that you could have the baby adopted.'

Helen

'A month after we started to try for a baby, I found out that I was pregnant! It came as a great shock because I hadn't thought things would happen so quickly. I think I was in a state of shock for quite a while because my pregnancy never seemed real to me until we went to the hospital for a routine scan when I was 20 weeks pregnant. The radiographer was an exceptionally nice woman who was obviously very good at her job. After scanning our baby for a while, she said that she thought she had found something wrong, but she didn't say immediately what her suspicions were. I was very frightened. When, after further scanning, she said that our little girl didn't have a right hand, I can only say that I felt immense relief that it was nothing worse!

'The radiographer said she would ask some specialist doctors to come and talk to us and we went off to the canteen while she made the necessary phone calls. Suddenly, I felt very, very protective towards my baby – and attached to her in a way that I hadn't been for the previous five months. I felt that I loved her immensely. I really didn't want anyone to tell me that this was a disaster and I certainly didn't want to consider an abortion.

'The care we had from the hospital was first class. When we went back to the ultrasound room to talk to the specialists, the radiographer said she would do another scan just to make sure that there was nothing else wrong. We were offered a further detailed scan at 28 weeks which we accepted although I was absolutely confident – I don't know why – that there wouldn't be any other problems.

'I told everyone – all my friends and all my family – about our little girl not having a hand. My Mum was tearful to begin with and shocked, but all my family were brilliant and we had lots of support from them. I'm so glad that everyone was able to prepare for the baby before she arrived. We did all the adjusting and grieving before she was born so that the actual birth was really marvellous, full of joy and excitement just as it should have been. If we hadn't known beforehand, we would have had to start our grieving when we already had Leanne with us. I think finding out while I was pregnant made a huge difference to the way we responded to her at birth and to our relationship with her ever since.

'After she was born, an obstetrician at the hospital said he admired the decision we had made. To begin with, I didn't know what he was talking about; then I realized that he was saying we could have had an abortion. To me, Leanne's problem is such a small one, I would never have thought of an abortion.

'We had a lot of support from the REACH organization after Leanne's birth and we continued to get excellent support from the hospital. We had the care of a very good paediatrician and were referred to a plastic surgeon. At the moment, Leanne doesn't wear an artificial hand and doesn't need one, but we know that when she is a little older, she may want to have another hand so that she can be like everyone else. We'll wait for her to make the decision.

'Leanne is now three years old. She has a close circle of friends who accept her completely. She's going to start nursery at the local school this year. As far as we are concerned, she is a normal little girl who does all the things normal little girls do. I know there may be some difficult times for her in the future, but we'll face those when we get there and I know we'll come through.'

Nicole

9

Antenatal Testing – Where Next?

It is probably true to say that there are, as yet, no ideal tests to enable women and their partners to find out whether their baby has Down's Syndrome or spina bifida or any other serious health problem. Whilst new tests are constantly being developed and it is now possible to know more about the unborn child than we have ever been able to know before, many people feel that the counselling which should accompany such testing is lagging far behind the new developments. Many women who have been through the mill of antenatal testing emerge shaken and disillusioned and question whether they were wise to have embarked on testing in the first place. A significant minority would now refuse all testing. On the other hand, those who want to keep women in control of their own fertility argue the case for a woman's right to know and to choose. Perhaps more time is needed to consider the human costs and ethical issues which are bound up in antenatal testing.

In the meantime, it is important for women to be helped and to help themselves to understand what is involved in having an antenatal test. Getting information and counselling can be difficult and this is especially true for women whose mother tongue is not English, or who are not sure of their dates or who do not book early in pregnancy for care.

A new National Screening Committee has now been set up to assess current screening programmes and to consider future developments. It is chaired by the Chief Medical Officer and both health professionals and users of health services are represented on the committee. One of its members, Pat Troop, commented recently:

> 'It is essential that screening programmes are assessed to draw up a balance sheet of benefit and harm before they are offered. It is also important for women to be given full information, so that they can choose whether or not to opt in or out of screening, or go ahead with any procedure or treatment offered.'
> (*Changing Childbirth Update*, June 1997, Issue 9, page 4)

In 1997, the National Childbirth Trust, the largest educational charity in the UK for parents with babies, carried out its own survey into women's feelings about antenatal testing. As a result of its research, the Trust suggested a series of guidelines to help parents get the best out of antenatal testing.

Guidelines for Parents

- ❑ Remember that you can choose whether to accept or refuse any test and whether or not to have an ultrasound scan.
- ❑ Ask as many questions as you need to before you make a decision about having tests for Down's Syndrome or spina bifida.
- ❑ If you decide not to have screening tests, you should not be put under pressure by people who have different views. You have

a right to exercise informed refusal as well as informed consent.

- ❏ It is not true that you can only have an amniocentesis if you would agree to a termination should your baby be found to have a disability.
- ❏ It's important to understand the difference between 'screening' tests which can only give you an estimate of the chance of your baby having a health problem and 'diagnostic' tests which give you a more definite answer.
- ❏ If you find out that your baby has Down's Syndrome or spina bifida, it may be helpful to contact self-help groups who can put you in touch with parents who have disabled children.
- ❏ Don't hesitate to go back to your hospital and ask for more information or support if you need to while you are waiting for results or when you are making decisions.
- ❏ You should have the chance to discuss antenatal testing with someone at your hospital who is a trained counsellor, or you should be referred to voluntary organizations which can provide counselling services if the hospital has no one available.

In the last resort, it may be up to us, as parents, to insist on the service we feel we need if antenatal testing is to enhance the experience of pregnancy rather than detract from it.

Suggestions for Further Reading

Introduction

Antenatal Screening and Abortion for Fetal Abnormality, edited by David Paintin, Chairman, Birth Control Trust. See Chapter 3 by Richard Lilford: 'Deciding What Screening Should Be Offered and How It Should Be Offered', pages 13–20. Published by Birth Control Trust, 1997.

Being Pregnant, Giving Birth by Mary Nolan. See Chapter 3: 'Antenatal Testing', pages 43–65. Published by National Childbirth Trust Publishing in collaboration with Thorsons, 1998.

Chapter 2

Cystic Fibrosis

Genetics, Carrier Tests and Tests during Pregnancy. Published by the Cystic Fibrosis Trust, 1995.

Screening for Cystic Fibrosis: Patient Guide. Published by Leeds Antenatal Screening Service, 1995.

HIV|AIDS

Understanding HIV Infection and AIDS. Published by The Terrence Higgins Trust, 1996.

Testing Issues: a booklet for people thinking of having an HIV test. Published by The Terrence Higgins Trust, 1996.

HIV/AIDS: Information for Women. Published by The Terrence Higgins Trust, 1996.

Positive Women: a guide to symptoms and treatments for women living with HIV and AIDS. Published by The Terrence Higgins Trust, 1997.

Pre-Eclampsia

Why Blood Pressure Is Checked in Pregnancy: A woman's guide to screening for pre-eclampsia. Published by Action on Pre-Eclampsia (APEC), 1996.

Sickle-Cell Disease

Sickle Cell: a guide for parents, guardians and families. Published by Sickle Cell Society, 1996.

Thalassaemia

All You Need to Know about Being a Carrier of Beta Thalassaemia. Published by the UK Thalassaemia Society, 1995.

Toxoplasmosis

Toxoplasmosis: you may never have heard of it – make sure your unborn baby doesn't. Published by The Toxoplasmosis Trust, undated.

Chapter 3

Down's Syndrome and Spina Bifida

Maternal Serum Screening for Down's Syndrome and Open Neural Tube Defects: General Information. Published by Antenatal Screening Service, St Bartholomew's and the Royal London School of Medicine and Dentistry, 1996.

Maternal Serum Screening for Down's Syndrome and Open Neural Tube Defects: Questions and Answers. Published by Antenatal Screening Service, St Bartholomew's and the Royal London School of Medicine and Dentistry, 1996.

Screening for Down's Syndrome: A Patient's Guide. Published by the Down's Syndrome Screening Service, Institute of Epidemiology, Leeds.

Chapter 4

Informed Choice for Women: Ultrasound scans: should you have one? Published by MIDIRS and the NHS Centre for Reviews and Dissemination, 1996.

Ultrasound? Unsound by Beverley A Lawrence Beech and Jean Robinson. Published by the Association for Improvements in the Maternity Services, 1996.

Chapter 6

Is My Baby Alright? by Christine Gosden, Kypros Nicolaides and Vanessa Whitting. Published by Oxford University Press, 1994.

Chapter 7

SATFA (Support Around Termination For Abnormality) newsletters. See Useful Addresses.

Chapter 9

The Stress of Tests in Pregnancy. A report by Rosemary Dodds of the National Childbirth Trust's antenatal screening survey of 2,700 women. Published by The National Childbirth Trust, 1997.

Useful Addresses

All these organizations have leaflets to help you think about antenatal testing and to enable you to find out more about the conditions which it is possible to diagnose during pregnancy. The ones marked with a star are voluntary organizations which also offer parent-to-parent support.

*Action on Pre-Eclampsia (APEC)

31–33 College Road
Harrow
Middlesex HA1 1EJ
Tel: 0181 863 3271

Antenatal Screening Service

(DEPM) Wolfson Institute of Preventive Medicine
St Bartholomew's & The Royal London School of Medicine
and Dentistry
Charterhouse Square
London EC1M 6BQ

Tel: 0171 982 6293/4
Fax: 0171 982 6290

*Association for Improvements in the Maternity Services

40 Kingswood Avenue
London NW6 6LS
Tel: 0181 960 5585

*Association for Spina Bifida and Hydrocephalus

ASBAH House
42 Park Road
Peterborough PE1 2UQ
Tel: 01733 555988

*Cystic Fibrosis Trust

11 London Road
Bromley
Kent BR1 1BY
Tel: 0181 464 7211

*Down's Syndrome Association

153–155 Mitcham Road
London SW17 9PG
Tel: 0181 682 4001

Harris Birthright Research Centre

King's College Hospital
Denmark Hill
London SE5 8RX
Tel: 0171 924 0894/0714

Leeds Antenatal Screening Service

26 Clarendon Road
Leeds LS2 9NZ
Tel: 0113 234 4013
Fax: 0113 233 6774

MIDIRS (Midwives' Information and Resource Service)

9 Elmdale Road
Clifton
Bristol BS8 1SL
Tel: 0800 581009

National Childbirth Trust

Alexandra House
Oldham Terrace
London W3 6NH
Tel: 0181 992 8637

*OSCAR (Organization for Sickle Cell Anaemia Research)

5 Lauderdale House
Goslin Way
Cowley Estate
London SW9 6JS
Tel: 0171 735 4166

*ParentAbility (Help for disabled parents – part of NCT)

National Childbirth Trust
Alexandra House
Oldham Terrace
London W3 6NH
Tel: 0181 992 2616 (9 a.m.–5 p.m.)

*Positively Women (Counselling and support for women with HIV and AIDS)

347 City Road
London EC1V 1LR
Tel: 0171 713 0222

*Reach (Charity for children with limb deficiencies)

12 Wilson Way
Earls Barton
Northants NN6 0NZ
Tel: 01604 811041

*Sickle Cell Society

54 Station Road
Harlesden
London NW10 4UB
Tel: 0181 961 7795

*Support Around Termination for Abnormality (SATFA)

29–30 Soho Square
London W1V 6JB
Tel: 0171 439 6124

*Terrence Higgins Trust (Services for people affected by HIV)

52–54 Grays Inn Road
London WC1X 8JU
Tel: 0171 831 0330

*Toxoplasmosis Trust

61 Collier Street
London N1 9BE
Tel: 0171 713 0599
E-mail: info@toxo.org.uk

*Women's Health (Information and support for women)

52 Featherstone Street
London EC1Y 8RT
Tel: 0171 251 6580

Other Voluntary Organizations Mentioned in this Book

*Relate

Herbert Gray College
Little Church Street
Rugby
Warwickshire CV21 3AP
Tel: 01788 573241

Index

markers 27–8

medical termination 74–8

MIDIRS (Midwives' Information and Resource Service) 104

Mifepristone (RU486) 74

miscarriage risk:
  and amniocentesis xviii–xix, 69
  and CVS 61–3, 64

National Childbirth Trust xxviii, 96, 104

National Screening Committee 96

nuchal translucency test xiv, xxi, 55–60

OSCAR (Organization for Sickle Cell Anaemia Research) 105

parents:
  and decision-making xx, xxviii–xxix, xxx, 38, 87, 96–7
  guidelines for 96–7

Patau's Syndrome 3

PatentAbility 105

perfect baby idea vii–viii

placenta, scanning 53

platelet level 9, 11

Positively Women 22, 105

pre-eclampsia 22–3

pregnancy diabetes 24

preparation:
  in decision-making xxix

for having tests xxix–xxx, 40–1

planning for sick or disabled baby x–xi, 93–4

questions:
  and amniocentesis 65
  prior to decision 96
  and ultrasound scans 52

Reach 105

reassurance x, xxv

Relate 82, 107

relaxation, method xxv

Remembrance Book 78

remembrances, of baby 76–7

results:
  getting xxvi, 35–6
  waiting for xxv–xxvi, 66–7, 97

rhesus factor 9–10

risk:
  and CVS 61, 62–3, 64
  and nuchal translucency test 60
  and screening tests xvi–xviii, 26, 34
  and ultrasound scans 43–4

rubella 9, 11–12

screen negative results xvi, xviii, xxvi, 28, 35, 37–8

screen positive results xvi, 28, 36–7

screening tests xiv–xxi, 26, 96–7

selective termination 79–80